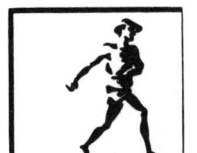

PREVIOUS BOOKS
BY WALTER McQUADE AND ANN AIKMAN
Stress

BY WALTER McQUADE
Cities Fit to Live In
Schoolhouse
The Joys She Chose (with Harry Middleton)

BY ANN AIKMAN
The Others

THE
LONG

A Revolutionary
New System
for Prolonging Your Life

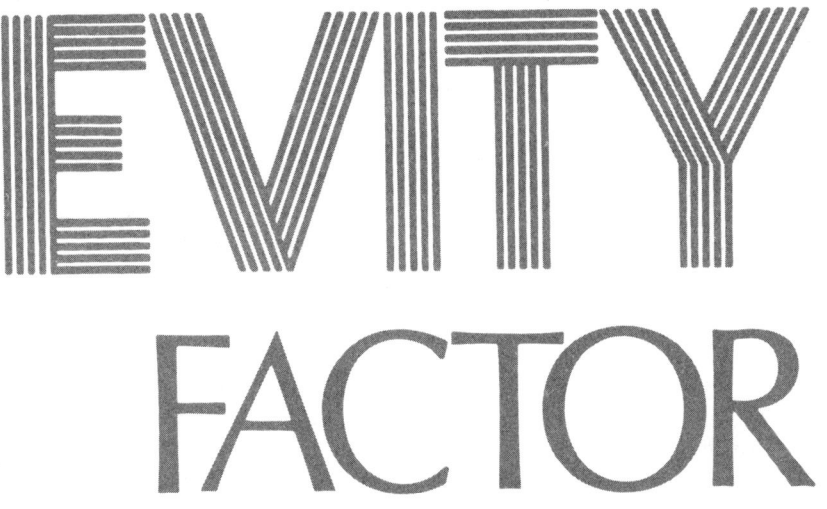

THE LONG-
EVITY
FACTOR

Walter McQuade
and Ann Aikman

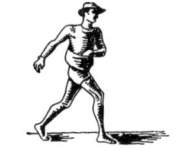

SIMON AND SCHUSTER
New York

Permission to reprint from the following is gratefully acknowledged:
Interhealth Questionnaire copyright © 1976 by Interhealth Medical Services, San Diego, CA, a division of Control Data Corporation's Life Extension Institute.
"How to Practice Prospective Medicine" copyright © 1970 and 1974 (second edition) by Health Hazard Appraisal, Inc.
Geller-Steele tables copyright © pending by Methodist Hospital, Indianapolis, IN.
"Your Lifestyle Profile" reprinted courtesy of Department of Health and Welfare, Ottawa, Canada.

Copyright © 1979 by Walter McQuade and Ann Aikman

All rights reserved
including the right of reproduction
in whole or in part in any form

Published by Simon and Schuster
A Division of Gulf & Western Corporation
Simon & Schuster Building
Rockefeller Center
1230 Avenue of the Americas
New York, New York 10020

Designed by Stanley S. Drate

Manufactured in the United States of America

1 2 3 4 5 6 7 8 9 10

Library of Congress Cataloging in Publication Data

McQuade, Walter.
   The longevity factor.

   Includes index.
   1. Health. 2. Health status indicators.
3. Longevity. 4. Life expectancy. I. Aikman, Ann, joint author. II. Title.
RA776.5.M26   613   79-10435

ISBN 0-671-24038-2

THE LONGEVITY FACTOR

Acknowledgments

Many specialists in preventive medicine have been helpful in charting this volume. Most particularly, the authors wish to thank Dr. Lewis C. Robbins and Dr. Charles M. Ross. It was Dr. Robbins who, as described in the text, originated the first workable health profiling method, Health Hazard Appraisal. He is also one of the founders of the Society of Prospective Medicine, a nationwide preventive medicine group which he currently serves as executive vice president. Dr. Robbins was most generous with his time, particularly in reviewing the details of the health profiling method, based on his own, in Chapter 17.

Dr. Ross, another dedicated physician, was president of the Society during the two years this book was under way, and also president and medical director of Interhealth Integrated Health Services of San Diego, a division of Control Data Corporation's Life Extension Institute. For his personal interest in the book, the many letters he wrote, the detailed advice he gave, and all the friendly hours we spent together, we will always cherish Charlie Ross.

Other members of the Society, now headed by Dr. Ronald G. Blankenbaker, were also helpful, among them: Dr. Edward Brethauer, Jr., Dr. Dean Davies, Sabina Dunton, Dr. Sam Fuenning,

ACKNOWLEDGMENTS

Harvey Geller, Norman Gesner, P. Lynn Hawkins, Dr. Bill Hettler, Dr. Ralph Hylinski, Dr. Harold Leppink, Dr. E. Dean Lovett, Lydia Ratcliff, Clark Robbins, Gregory Steele, William Thompson, Jr., and H. Lynn Warner.

The concept of this book first emerged in conversations with Dr. John P. McCann, medical board chairman of the Life Extension Institute. Throughout, Dr. McCann supplied us with ideas and information, as did numerous members of his staff, particularly Dr. Donald C. Kent, Lloyd Shewchuck, Dolores Floss, and Marilyn Zeller.

On the Interhealth staff in San Diego, Russell O. French, Susan Macartney, Dorothy Barr, and Sunny Christiansen were both patient and helpful.

Dr. Jack Hall of Methodist Hospital in Indianapolis reviewed sections of the book and provided useful advice and permissions. Others with special knowledge in the prevention field who rendered important assistance: Dr. Herbert Spiegel, Dr. Joan Ullyot, Dr. Robert J. Fallat, Jacquelyn Rogers, Dr. Jon Rogers, Jane Fullarton, Tony DiMelfi, and Don Samuels.

We are very grateful to the numerous individuals interviewed for the personal sketches in Part II—just nine could be used because of space limitations. They gave us many hours of their time, and abundant insights into the problems of prevention in people's personal lives.

Thanks go to the executives of Time, Inc., particularly to Robert Lubar, Managing Editor of *Fortune* magazine, for granting a leave of absence to one of the authors to work full time on the book.

Finally, we give thanks to two expert researchers, Louise Campbell and Mary Elizabeth Allison, who helped in our investigation of certain materials, and to Molly McQuade, who typed the original manuscript with such dispatch. Only the authors, however, are responsible for the interpretations and opinions expressed in the book.

Contents

ACKNOWLEDGMENTS   9

Part I

1 HOW ARE YOU?   15

2 ONE SUSAN JOHNSON   18

3 DOCTORS, DEATH, AND PEOPLE   25

4 THE POSTPONABLE DISEASES   33

Part II

5 AGE 40—TIME TO GROW UP:
   Donald Hanson, Alcoholic   55

6 QUITTING WHILE YOU'RE AHEAD:
   Laura Blake, Smoker   72

7 QUITTING AFTER IT'S TOO LATE:
   Eugene Howell, Smoker   85

8 TRYING:
   Lucille Meeker, Overeater   101

9 A STRENUOUS MENU:
　　Ed Solomon, Angina Patient　　　　　　　　*116*

10 BACK FROM SELF-DESTRUCTION:
　　Kathleen Mooney, Alcoholic　　　　　　　　*128*

11 CHANGING ACROSS THE BOARD:
　　Jack Kodaly, "Normal" Health　　　　　　　*148*

12 OUTRANGING THE AGE TABLES:
　　Emily Eastman, 85　　　　　　　　　　　　*159*

13 THE VERY BEST OF HEALTH:
　　Jim Garro, Disturbing Family History　　　　*172*

Part III

14 CHANGING HABITS　　　　　　　　　　　*181*

Part IV

15 YOUR OWN HEALTH PROFILE:
　　The Short Form　　　　　　　　　　　　　*197*

16 YOUR OWN HEALTH PROFILE:
　　Computer-Assisted　　　　　　　　　　　　*201*

17 YOUR OWN HEALTH PROFILE:
　　Do It Yourself　　　　　　　　　　　　　　*223*

　　APPENDIX A　　　　　　　　　　　　　　*279*

　　APPENDIX B　　　　　　　　　　　　　　*285*

　　INDEX　　　　　　　　　　　　　　　　　*291*

PART III

1
HOW ARE YOU?

The patient comes in for his annual checkup. His doctor examines him, then sits him down and begins urging him to amend his ways.

"Oh, you're right," concedes the patient. "Of course you're right. Still, you didn't find anything really wrong, did you? I feel okay. I don't seem to have any symptoms."

"Not yet," the doctor answers quietly.

The patient goes away. No doubt about it, he's troubled. At home he takes out a cigarette and just looks at it for a moment or two.

Then he lights the cigarette, downs a couple of martinis, and ingests a cholesterol-rich dinner.

After that he feels like himself again.

Smokers can't seem to quit smoking. The overweight can't stick to their diets. People suffering from edema don't like the looks of the bags under their eyes, but blink away doing anything about them. Sedentary types can't make themselves come home from the office and do calisthenics for half an hour; they won't even walk home from the commuter station.

Perhaps the reason is that all of us are born mortal, and we learn to accept this fact quite early in life. *Who wants to live forever?* we ask ourselves.

It isn't eternity that we need, but time—enough years in our lives so we can accomplish the things that are important to us. We also want sufficient good health during these years to do the same. And we hope, when our time does come, for a quick, "easy" death. Medical science, we like to believe, will solve these matters for us.

Science has been most successful with the first of them—statistical longevity. Smallpox, typhoid, tuberculosis, and the other infectious scourges that struck down so many of our ancestors in the prime of life have all been virtually conquered. Today more and more people can expect to live into reasonable old age—the seventies and eighties.

The results, however, are not so happy. Hospitals and nursing homes are still full, and the afflictions that people suffer are in some ways harder to bear than those of a hundred years ago. Heart disease, cancer, strokes, cirrhosis, arthritis, emphysema; these are typical of the so-called chronic diseases, lingering, crippling, painful, impervious to any known vaccine or antibiotic. And some of them strike young.

The best way to "cure" these degenerative diseases is to prevent them, ahead of time. The catch is that the person who does the preventing is not the doctor or the scientist, but you. True, techniques have been developed by groups such as Alcoholics Anonymous, Weight Watchers, and Smokenders to help people change habits. But first they must want to change. A recent device addresses itself to the problem, and that is what this book is principally about.

The device goes by various names: Health Hazard Appraisal, Health Risk Analysis, Health Risk Profile. We will assign it a generic name, health profiling.

Health profiling starts with a questionnaire asking you

the details of your past and current health, your personal habits, your family medical history, and your vital statistics in blood pressure and the like. The resulting information is submitted to calculation (most easily performed by computer, but you can also do it yourself with a pencil and pad of paper) in a formula which weighs you against an average American of your category in age and race—for example, male, black, 40 years of age. Then back comes the result, a detailed statement informing you just what you can expect in terms of your health—particularly in terms of fatal disease—over the period of the coming ten years.

After that, the health profile goes on to tell you how your prospects can be improved if you decide to change the way you live—by bringing your blood pressure down, as one example, which practically all hypertensive people can do these days.

In short, the health profile answers the commonplace question that heads this chapter: How are you? How are you *really?*

Then it shows you what you can do about it.

2
ONE SUSAN JOHNSON

In the final section of this book you will learn how to construct your own health profile. Meantime, let's see how the device works, by looking over the shoulder of one Susan Johnson. She exists, although that is not her true name.

Susan was divorced about a year ago, and has a fifteen-year-old son at home. She is somewhat overweight, smokes and drinks more than most (particularly during her recent marital crisis), and drives about 12,000 miles a year, usually without a seat belt. One day Susan fills out a questionnaire and sends it off with a blood sample to a preventive medicine laboratory in San Diego. Several weeks later back comes an envelope marked "confidential," containing her Health Risk Profile, the laboratory's name for its profiling method. She opens it and begins reading. (A slightly condensed version of Susan's health profile appears at the end of this chapter.)

"An average white woman your age," she reads, "has 2,852 chances per 100,000 of dying in the next ten years; your risks are 54 percent greater than the average."

This is clear-cut language, but in case Susan misses the point, the same truth is also expressed in terms of years. Though chronologically Susan is 40, the state of her health makes her the equivalent of 46—while she *could* be, with a little effort, the equivalent of 39.

The report next summarizes what steps Susan can take to improve her odds, and tells her how many years or fractions of years each revision will give her. For instance, she will gain 1.9 years if she stops smoking, .3 years if she gets her weight back to normal.

After that the Health Risk Profile lists, in order of probability, the specific afflictions that could kill Susan Johnson in the coming decade, enumerating in detail the circumstances that make each a possibility. Once again, three figures are given—the *average risk* for people of her sex, race, and age; her own *current risk* based on the ways she tests medically, her family history, and the way she has chosen to live; and, finally, her *achievable risk*. These figures are represented by numbers, and emphasized graphically by rows of black dots.

Susan goes down the list until she comes to the end. Then she reads it over a second time, frowning slightly. She lays it down. At last she picks it up and begins to peruse it again. *Yes, but* . . . her mind keeps murmuring.

Yes, but a daiquiri before lunch relaxes me.
Yes, but my father was a smoker, and he lived to be 81.

The health profile doesn't argue these matters with her. It just keeps giving her back the statistical probabilities, every time she picks up her printout.

Arteriosclerotic heart disease, for instance. Her chances of suffering a fatal heart attack in the next ten years are 2.6 times the average for a woman her age.

And cirrhosis of the liver. That's an alcoholic's disease, and Susan's no alcoholic. Yet look at her statistics! If she stopped drinking completely, she'd reduce her risk from that unpleasant disease to one-twelfth of what it is now. It's hard for Susan to get those rows of extra dots out of her head.

She also keeps thinking of her age. Only a few weeks ago Susan turned 40, a change that's been depressing her mildly. Now she discovers she *could* be, in terms of her health, back in her thirties again—she could be only 39. But instead, because of the way she lives, she's really, in effect, six years *older* than 40; 46 is more than halfway to 50.

Susan is morose, and not only because of her personal statistics. Behind them lies a truth, not part of her way of thinking, which now, suddenly, she has to come to grips with: *I, Susan Johnson, am sole proprietor of my body. If I treat it with care and respect, it will reciprocate, treating me well, lasting a long time. If I don't, I must pay the consequences.*

* * *

Note: In the health profile of Susan Johnson below, and in all other health profiles, the lower the numerical point rating the better. For example, in arteriosclerotic heart disease, Susan's rating of .7 on cholesterol means she is running a risk, so far as cholesterol is concerned, of .7 times the average for people in her category, or 30 percent below that of the average white woman her age; whereas her 2.1 rating on smoking means that her risk (so far as smoking is concerned) is 2.1 times the average, or 210 percent higher.

The black dots give a graphic representation of proportionate risk: 10 dots signifies an average risk; 5 would signify a risk half the average; and 20 would signify a risk two times the average.

ONE SUSAN JOHNSON

HEALTH RISK PROFILE

Susan Johnson, age 40, white.

Age in terms of present health, 46.

Achievable health age, 39.

An average white woman your age has 2,852 chances of dying per 100,000 in the next ten years; your risks are 54% greater than the average. You can, however, reduce these risks by 42%.

FACTORS OFFERING THE GREATEST REDUCTION IN RISK:	THE NUMBER OF YEARS TO BE GAINED BY ALTERING THOSE FACTORS:
Drinking	3.0 years
Smoking	1.9 years
Exercise	.4 year
Weight	.3 year
Other Factors	1.4 years
Total	7.0 years

Your risks of death within the next ten years in descending importance:

1. ARTERIOSCLEROTIC HEART DISEASE (heart attack)

AVERAGE RISK	308 ●●●●●●●●●●
YOUR CURRENT RISK	795 ●●●●●●●●●●●●●●●●●●●●●●●●●●
YOUR ACHIEVABLE RISK	160 ●●●●●

INDICATORS OF RISK	RISK RATING	WAYS TO REDUCE RISK	RISK RATING
Current blood pressure 120/70	.4		
Current cholesterol 203	.7	Cholesterol 180 or less	.6
Diabetes—none	1.0		
Exercise—sedentary	1.4	Exercise—vigorous	1.0

THE LONGEVITY FACTOR

HEALTH RISK PROFILE (cont.)

Family history of early heart deaths—one parent	1.2		
Smoker—2 packs per day	2.1	Not smoking	.9
Weight 160 lbs.	1.3	Reduce to 119 lbs. or less	1.0
History of abnormal electrocardiogram—none	1.0		
Current triglycerides 234	1.3	Triglycerides 151 or less	1.1

Excessive stress may increase risk. Exact risk factor not yet available.

2. BREAST CANCER

AVERAGE RISK	342 ●●●●●●●●●●
YOUR CURRENT RISK	581 ●●●●●●●●●●●●●●●●●●
YOUR ACHIEVABLE RISK	342 ●●●●●●●●●●

INDICATORS OF RISK	RISK RATING	WAYS TO REDUCE RISK	RISK RATING
Family history of breast cancer—yes Monthly self-examination—no Yearly exam by physician—yes Yearly mammography—no	1.7	Monthly self-examination Yearly mammography	1.0

3. MOTOR VEHICLE ACCIDENTS

AVERAGE RISK	93 ●●●●●●●●●●
YOUR CURRENT RISK	456 ●●
YOUR ACHIEVABLE RISK	37 ●●●●

ONE SUSAN JOHNSON

INDICATORS OF RISK	RISK RATING	WAYS TO REDUCE RISK	RISK RATING
Alcohol consumption—25 to 40 drinks per week	5.0	No drinks before driving	.5
Mileage yearly as driver or passenger—12,000	1.0		
Seat belt use—25% to 74% of time	.9	Use seat belts always	.8

4. LUNG CANCER

AVERAGE RISK	149 ●●●●●●●●●●
YOUR CURRENT RISK	447 ●●●●●●●●●●●●●●●●●●●●●●●●●●●●●●
YOUR ACHIEVABLE RISK	358 ●●●●●●●●●●●●●●●●●●●●●●●●●

INDICATORS OF RISK	RISK RATING	WAYS TO REDUCE RISK	RISK RATING
Smoker—2 packs per day	3.0	Not smoking	2.4
		Remain stopped 6 years	.6

5. CIRRHOSIS OF THE LIVER

AVERAGE RISK	170 ●●●●●●●●●●●
YOUR CURRENT RISK	425 ●●●●●●●●●●●●●●●●●●●●●●●●●●●
YOUR ACHIEVABLE RISK	34 ●●

INDICATORS OF RISK	RISK RATING	WAYS TO REDUCE RISK	RISK RATING
Alcohol consumption—25 to 40 drinks per week	2.5	Not drinking	.2
Liver function test normal	1.0		

Susan Johnson's health profile then evaluates her other risks in order of danger: suicide, stroke, cancer of the ovary, cancer of the large intestine and rectum, and cancer of the cervix. On all of these, she scores average or better for her age group. Her complete profile is reproduced in Appendix B at the end of this volume.

3
DOCTORS, DEATH, AND PEOPLE

What Susan Johnson has just come up against is the basic concept of modern preventive medicine.

Centuries ago, sickness was regarded as fate or, perhaps more often, as a visitation from God to punish us for our wickedness. Then, as we gradually learned something of the mechanics of disease, we began placing our well-being in the hands of professional doctors. There it remains, for most of us, today. We wait until we fall ill, then we go to a doctor, and, in effect, purchase some health. Otherwise, we rarely think about the matter. Health isn't our business. It's the business of the medical profession.

Thus the idea that the individual person bears responsibility for his own physical condition is relatively new. But it is an idea that is spreading, particularly as medical research probes further into the causes of human disease. Susan's grandparents never heard of cholesterol, and considered an extra 20 pounds of weight to be a sign of good health. Today people know more—and can prevent more.

In addition, the traditional approach to medical care is running into serious financial problems. Take Susan's risk of heart disease, elevated to 2½ times the average by her habits in smoking, eating, and exercise. If Susan changes these habits, she can improve her prospects without spending a cent. But if she goes on living as she has been, and the statistics catch up with her, she could be in for an expensive time indeed. Death is not all she must fear: for each person who dies of heart disease annually, approximately seven are disabled by it. Their costs are borne not only by themselves, but by the rest of society, in the form of medical insurance premiums, government subsidies, and the like. Medical care is now the third biggest business in the United States (after only building and agriculture), costing an estimated $205 billion per year. This is more than 9 percent of the gross national product, compared with only 5.9 percent (or $40 billion) in 1965.

Recently a few prominent physicians such as the late Dr. John Knowles, president of the Rockefeller Foundation, have begun prodding their fellow citizens, and prodding their fellow physicians, too, toward preventive medicine. In a 1977 survey published in *Daedalus* magazine, titled "Doing Better and Feeling Worse: Health in the United States," Knowles wryly described American society as "a credit-minded culture which does it now and pays for it later, whether in drinking and eating or in buying cars and houses. . . . Over 99 percent of us are born healthy and suffer premature death and disability only as a result of personal misbehavior and environmental conditions."

The solution is obvious: prevention. Yet Knowles pointed out that of the billions of dollars spent on health in this country annually, less than 3 percent goes to disease prevention and control. Doctors themselves, he said, are not interested in prevention because "the intellectual, emotional, and financial rewards of the present system are too great." As for the general public, it prefers to think that good health is a job for the doctor, not the patient. Knowles said, "The idea of a 'right' to health should be replaced by the idea of an individual moral obligation to preserve one's own health," but he was gloomy about the chances for such a change in attitude.

One who shares Knowles' basic view, if not his pessimism, is Dr. Lewis C. Robbins, a long-time preventive medicine specialist and the man who, back in the 1950s, developed the first profiling technique, Health Hazard Appraisal. In his long career in medicine, Robbins has exemplified the kind of preventive medicine approach that Knowles and a few other doctors, economists, and political leaders say we need so badly. That approach is a combination of science and sociology.

Robbins, a thoroughgoing midwesterner, was born in Indianapolis, and was pointed early toward a doctor's life. As an eight-year-old he began raising guinea pigs for a neighboring doctor for seriological testing. Then, as a boy scout, he specialized in first aid and, by the time he was 19, landed the job of heading up the first-aid crews scattered among the crowds who attended the annual Indianapolis 500. Each year as many as 150,000 people came to the race to sit for many hours under May skies, devour various hawkers' foods, and, above all, consume copious quantities of beer and bourbon whiskey. Young Robbins was only a premedical student when he got the job, but by the time he left it he was a full-fledged physician, graduated from Indiana University in 1935.

He went on to the Johns Hopkins Medical School for postgraduate work in public health, then joined the federal Public Health Service, beginning a life that was to shift him, like a peripatetic army officer, between stations as varied as Wichita Falls, Texas, and Saigon, Indochina. Many physicians at the time took a somewhat snobbish view of preventive medicine specialists, and some still do. This has never bothered Robbins. "I wanted to save lives," he says, "in great numbers."

Following World War II, his specialty began to emerge and he attained a certain prominence. The U.S. Congress decided that something had to be done about heart disease, and pressed the Public Health Service to take action. In 1947 the Service sent Robbins and another physician to a small Massachusetts city to set up an investigation of heart disease. This became the famous Framingham study, perhaps the single most definitive public health project ever undertaken in pursuit of a specific disease, and one that is still going on today. What has been learned so far is that the best way to stave off coronaries and other cardiovascular troubles is to live right, chiefly through controlling weight, deemphasizing fat in the diet, not smoking, and taking regular exercise. In 1957 Robbins was named to head a Public Health Service effort against the second most dreaded killer, cancer, and it was then that he began to develop health profiling. In 1968 he returned to Methodist Hospital in Indianapolis and enlisted the interest of other physicians on the staff, most prominently Dr. Jack H. Hall, vice president for medical education. The State of Indiana helped support their work with a series of grants. In the past decade more than 100,000 individual Health Hazard Appraisals have been processed, and the program has been computerized.

In 1970 Robbins and Hall also published a book to teach health profiling to family physicians, *How to Practice Prospective Medicine,* and both are founding members of a national organization, the Society of Prospective Medicine, which devotes itself to the technique of health profiling and to preventive medicine generally, and is growing rapidly.

* * *

Health profiling is so recent that scientific studies of its effectiveness have only begun. Major among them at present is an evaluation being conducted at the University of

Arizona in Tucson, where Sabina Dunton, a public health expert, is profiling faculty members and their spouses, and also using health profiles in a preventive medicine drive in ten small Arizona communities. There will be follow-ups, control groups, and all the other paraphernalia of modern scientific testing, supported by a four-year grant from the W. K. Kellogg Foundation.

Blue Cross, the medical insurance company, is running a study too, underwriting the cost of profiling for the entire faculty of Palomar College in San Diego (as well as using profiling in its own staff medical plan in areas of the Midwest). Meanwhile, Southern California Blue Cross has added health profiling to its list of compensable benefits.

Of completed studies, the most thorough to date probably remains the test run in 1974 at the NASA center in Moffet Field, California, by three health professionals: Joseph LaDou, M.D., John N. Sherwood, M.D., and Lewis Hughes, Ph.D. Under their surveillance, 488 NASA personnel participated in a program of annual free medical examinations, including blood testing, chest X-rays, and electrocardiograms, plus a comprehensive profiling questionnaire which, with the physical statistics, was fed into a computer. Afterward, the results were explained to each employee in a private session with a doctor.

Within a year the three medics picked, at random, 107 of the people examined earlier, and another profile was run on each. At the time of the first profiling, the average risk age had been 49, about a month worse than the actual chronological ages. But by the second round the participants had improved 1.4 years on the average, to set their new risk ages well *below* their actual ages. In a few months of effort, these 107 relatively healthy people had earned themselves a total of almost 150 years of extra predicted life.

More informal tests, meanwhile, are performed with frequency—including a recent one in Salt Lake City, where

H. Lynn Warner, of the Utah State Division of Health, decided to introduce profiling to a group of her staff professionals, the majority of them nurses. With some backing from HEW, she asked professional consultants to come in, explain the profiling questionnaire, take blood samples, test them, and deliver computerized profiles to the seventy-five people enrolled.

There was an added feature in Ms. Warner's program, however. After the printouts were distributed and their contents absorbed, the participants were invited to choose a habit they wanted to change and then sign a contract drawn up by an attending lawyer. The degree of habit change was to be specified in each contract. Smokers, for example, might elect to drop the habit entirely, or to cut down by a certain percentage. If exercise was the goal, both the type of activity and the time to be spent on it were stated.

The six most frequently pledged changes were:

1. Getting more exercise
2. Losing weight
3. Wearing seat belts oftener
4. Reducing intake of fats and cholesterol
5. Undertaking periodic medical checkups
6. Controlling stress

To help get started, participants were all offered individual counseling sessions.

Six months later the results were assessed. Success was substantial. Of the 78 pledges to get more exercise (the number was so large because some participants contracted for more than one type of exercise), no fewer than 55 were completely fulfilled, with another 23 fairly good stabs at performing. Of 60 who had sworn to lose weight, 25 hit their targets, an extraordinarily high proportion in weight loss. More than 80 percent of those who promised to get a medical checkup did so. Of seven who decided to cut out or modify their smoking, three succeeded completely and another four partially. And three out of five managed to reduce their blood pressure. Surprisingly, attempts to increase the use of seat belts, which sounds so easy, were only 50 percent successful.

Down the long list of resolves were some wistful contracts; of the two people who had promised themselves to "keep smiling" only one succeeded. But the man who pledged to run a marathon did so, and another exerciser worked himself up to a 250-mile bicycle trip. Lynn Warner herself signed no contracts, but after six months she bought a pair of Adidas running shoes and at last report was jogging five miles a day.

Meanwhile, Dr. Lew Robbins, the inventor of profiling, feels sanguine about the future: though he's been in prevention all his life and knows the problems, the truth, he says, is so obvious. Robbins has a chart he likes to draw to demonstrate the natural history of a degenerative disease such as lung cancer over the course of a given person's lifetime. It goes like this:

1. *Birth. Your risk is close to zero.*
2. *You become vulnerable to a precursor (e.g., smoking).*
3. *You start smoking. Your risk begins to rise slowly.*
4. Signs *of disease, unknown to you, begin to develop, such as changes in lung tissue. Your risk rises further.*
5. *You develop* symptoms *that you can feel—cough, chest discomfort, and so on. Your risk goes higher still.*
6. *Disability. Your risk of death from lung cancer is now between 90 and 95 percent.*
7. *Death.*

The length of time between stage 3, when you first start smoking, and stage 6, disability, can vary from twenty years to forty or more. But with each year you continue smoking, your risk rises inexorably.

The question, says Robbins, is this: At what stage should you intervene? Conventional medicine intervenes at stage 6, employing surgery, chemotherapy, and other painful and costly measures; at best, it saves one out of ten patients.

Robbins wants to intervene at stage 2 and save everybody.

4
THE POSTPONABLE DISEASES

When Lew Robbins first looked into the possibilities of health profiling, he had a young statistician on his staff, Harvey Geller, who soon joined the profiling project. It became Geller's task to study causes of death, based on nationwide mortality figures, and break them down into age groups. Later he broke them down by sex and race as well, sorted them into tables, and produced what came to be called the Geller tables.* These tables are basic not only to health profiling techniques, but to preventive medicine generally. They contain some surprises. For example, if you are a black male aged 20, your likeliest cause of death in the decade ahead is murder; if you are a white female of 30, it is suicide.

At the end of this chapter you will find the most recent set of cause-of-death tables printed in their entirety. You will need the tables later to compute your own health profile. But meantime they can tell you a good deal about your-

---

* They are now known as the Geller-Steele tables, because they represent a continuing collaboration of Geller with Gregory Steele of the University of South Florida.

self and about the society you live in. You might take a break right now and run an eye down the lists (see pages 39–52).

These are the causes of death in America today. Not diphtheria and typhoid. Rarely tuberculosis. But over and over again, with grim monotony, arteriosclerotic heart disease; stroke; cancer of the lung, of the breast, of the large intestine and rectum. Notice that it is not only the elderly who succumb. Heart disease kills U.S. males at an annual rate of one per hundred as early as age 40, and the rate rises sharply with increased age. Cancer kills one per hundred females starting at age 45.

Then there are our "lesser" scourges: cirrhosis; auto accidents; homicide and suicide; respiratory diseases like pneumonia, emphysema, and chronic bronchitis; diabetes.

* * *

Let's take these threats one by one and see what it is that we're doing wrong:

Cardiovascular disease. This includes heart attacks and strokes, and both are common among people who

1. Smoke cigarettes
2. Have high blood pressure
3. Have high levels of serum cholesterol in their blood
4. Are overweight
5. Get little exercise
6. Have an adverse family history (cardiovascular disease in one or both parents)

Your risk rises further still if you suffer from diabetes, especially if it is not under treatment.

Cancer. Today we know that many types of human malignancy are caused by carcinogens—chemicals and other irritants you may happen to eat, breathe, or absorb through

THE POSTPONABLE DISEASES

your skin. Cigarette smoke, alcohol, benzene, the nitrates in your bacon, the asbestos in your brake linings, ordinary sunshine—these are a few of the thousands of known carcinogens * which, added together, help account for 90 percent of all cancers, according to the National Cancer Institute.

Does this mean that perhaps 90 percent of all cancers could be *prevented,* simply by avoiding the carcinogens causing them? Theoretically, yes. But progress is disappointing. Manufacturers who use carcinogenic chemicals in their products tend to resist change, and government agencies seem reluctant to pressure them really forcefully. Meanwhile, new chemicals keep coming out of the laboratories at a steady clip. Some are safe and some aren't: we won't be certain for years because the hard evidence—actual malignancy in real human beings—is so slow to develop. Cigarette smoking first became widespread in the early 1920s, but it wasn't till the forties that lung cancer increased significantly, and it took even longer for medical men to recognize the reason. By 1964, when the Surgeon General finally issued his warning, 65 million Americans were hooked by the smoking habit.

New chemicals can, of course, be tried out on animals with relatively quick results, but this kind of evidence is usually contested by business interests and often fails to persuade regulatory commissions as well. Sodium nitrite is used as a preservative and coloring agent for many different meat products; it is perfectly legal, although when heated it causes the development of nitrosamines, which are known to produce tumors in laboratory animals.

Cirrhosis of the liver is an affliction of heavy drinkers; its

---

* At present, 2,415 substances are officially listed as carcinogens by the U.S. government's Occupational Safety and Health Administration.

35

incidence in nondrinkers is minuscule. Once diagnosed, cirrhosis can usually be halted if the patient stops drinking. Many victims, however, do not or cannot stop, and the disease ends in death each year for 16 out of every 100,000 Americans, most of them between the ages of 50 and 60. This figure is up from 11.8 per 100,000 in 1916.

In the United Kingdom, incidentally, the cirrhosis death rate is *down* by more than two-thirds during the same period—because of extremely high taxes on liquor, it is thought.

Motor vehicle accidents, the leading cause of death among young people, are closely linked to alcohol consumption and increasingly to other drugs as well, from marijuana to seemingly innocent tranquilizers. In 1976 alcohol played a part in half the traffic deaths in the nation; the figure for marijuana was 11 percent that same year in the State of California. The other big consideration in accidents is, of course, exposure, as measured in mileage, either at the wheel or as a passenger. A farm supervisor in Bakersfield, California, for example, will have a traffic death risk that is abnormal not so much because he drinks—though he probably does—but because he drives 80,000 to 100,000 miles a year.

Seat belts could save more years of life than all the medicines sold, but fewer than 20 percent of Americans use them regularly.

Suicide and homicide. Preventable? In a sense. If you are subject to moods of serious depression, a timely nudge might induce you to seek help rather than drift downward into the vortex of suicide statistics. Or if on occasion you have used violence to get what you want, and you sometimes carry a weapon, knowledge of the statistical consequences could lead you to change.

Respiratory diseases. These depend almost exclusively

THE POSTPONABLE DISEASES

on what you breathe. Clean country air? Cigarette smoke? Asbestos fibers? Of these, asbestos fibers are by far the most damaging, but smoking causes more illness simply because it is so widespread. Even with the occupational diseases—black lung, asbestosis—it is the smokers who are stricken first; cigarettes multiply the effects of the other contaminants.

Some smokers get emphysema, a permanent and incurable lung affliction. Chronic bronchitis, asthma, and pneumonia are also common in people who breathe unhealthy air—the single broadest cause of which, again, is cigarettes.

Diabetes. A major medical breakthrough came in 1922 when it was discovered that once-fatal forms of diabetes could be controlled by insulin medication. Today countless diabetics prolong their lives for many years through a closely balanced mix of injections, diet, and exercise. Ultimately, however, more Americans die of the disease now than back in 1900. This is because there are greater numbers of diabetics today—perhaps 4 million among us, of whom half have not even been diagnosed. Diabetes also kills indirectly, by causing heart disease and stroke. It runs in families, and is most likely to strike overweight, sedentary people who have a fondness for sweets. In 1975, the most recent year for which records are available, Americans consumed 87.5 pounds of refined sugar per capita, a very high figure.

Cardiovascular disease, cancer, cirrhosis of the liver, motor vehicle accidents, suicide, homicide, respiratory diseases, diabetes; we cannot cure these health problems, and in most cases we cannot even prevent them 100 percent. What we can do is postpone their advent into our lives. Let's call them the *postponables*.

And let's see how they are postponed, by going down the list once more. What are the major factors that crop up again and again in these causes of death?

- Poor eating habits: in cardiovascular disease and diabetes
- Insufficient exercise: also in cardiovascular disease and diabetes
- Smoking: in cardiovascular disease, respiratory diseases, and some forms of cancer
- High alcohol consumption: in cirrhosis, motor vehicle accidents, and some forms of cancer (also, incidentally, in pneumonia, still a prominent respiratory disease)
- Environmental exposure: particularly in cancer and respiratory diseases

There are minor threads too, such as use of seat belts, but these are the five major ones that keep repeating themselves. Change just one of them, and you automatically lower your risks for several different causes of death.

Susan Johnson's health profile shows she is taking risks in four of these five areas. How about you?

Your profile (see Chapters 15 through 17) will provide the answer. Study it.

Then start studying the changes you want to make.

Death in the United States

There are close to 4,000 causes of death listed by the U.S. Public Health Service, but fewer than 50 take by far the greatest number of lives. The Geller-Steele tables extend from age 5 through 74, in five-year groupings of males and females, blacks and whites; the tables predict, for people in each category, the probability of dying in the next ten years.

THE POSTPONABLE DISEASES

WHITE MALES, AGE 5–9	PER 100,000
1. Motor vehicle accidents	112
2. Drownings	46
3. Leukemia	31
4. Accidents with firearms	18
5. Accidents involving machines (excluding cars)	17
6. Brain cancer	15
7. Fire	15
8. Congenital heart defects	15
9. Pneumonia	12
10. Homicide	10
All other causes combined	179

WHITE FEMALES, AGE 5–9	PER 100,000
1. Motor vehicle accidents	66
2. Leukemia	24
3. Congenital circulatory defects	14
4. Brain cancer	12
5. Fire	12
6. Drownings	12
7. Pneumonia	11
8. Cystic fibrosis	8
9. Stroke	6
10. Hydrocephalus	6
All other causes combined	129

BLACK MALES, AGE 5–9	PER 100,000
1. Motor vehicle accidents	150
2. Drownings	114
3. Homicide	32
4. Fire	31
5. Accidents with firearms	27
6. Leukemia	21
7. Pneumonia	19
8. Brain cancer	16
9. Anemias	11
10. Accidents involving machines (excluding cars)	9
All other causes combined	240

BLACK FEMALES, AGE 5–9	PER 100,000
1. Motor vehicle accidents	77
2. Fire	36
3. Drownings	22
4. Homicide	22
5. Brain cancer	15
6. Leukemia	15
7. Pneumonia	15
8. Anemias	10
9. Congenital circulatory defects	10
10. Hydrocephalus	9
All other causes combined	169

THE LONGEVITY FACTOR

WHITE MALES, AGE 10–14	PER 100,000
1. Motor vehicle accidents	400
2. Drownings	72
3. Suicide	70
4. Homicide	46
5. Accidents involving machines (excluding cars)	35
6. Accidents with firearms	31
7. Poisonings	24
8. Leukemia	24
9. Pneumonia	14
10. Falls	14
All other causes combined	290

WHITE FEMALES, AGE 10–14	PER 100,000
1. Motor vehicle accidents	146
2. Suicide	20
3. Homicide	19
4. Leukemia	16
5. Congenital circulatory defects	12
6. Pneumonia	11
7. Drownings	10
8. Brain cancer	9
9. Poisonings	9
10. Stroke	8
All other causes combined	170

BLACK MALES, AGE 10–14	PER 100,000
1. Homicide	325
2. Motor vehicle accidents	214
3. Drownings	167
4. Accidents with firearms	49
5. Suicide	31
6. Poisonings	22
7. Leukemia	22
8. Pneumonia	21
9. Accidents involving machines (excluding cars)	19
10. Congenital circulatory defects	15
All other causes combined	405

BLACK FEMALES, AGE 10–14	PER 100,000
1. Homicide	99
2. Motor vehicle accidents	69
3. Drownings	24
4. Pneumonia	19
5. Fire	18
6. Complications of pregnancy and abortions	16
7. Suicide	16
8. Poisonings	14
9. Leukemia	13
10. Stroke	12
All other causes combined	280

THE POSTPONABLE DISEASES

WHITE MALES, AGE 15–19	PER 100,000
1. Motor vehicle accidents	691
2. Suicide	189
3. Homicide	120
4. Drownings	82
5. Poisonings	59
6. Accidents involving machines (excluding cars)	59
7. Accidents with firearms	34
8. Falls	26
9. Leukemia	21
10. Water transportation accidents	20
All other causes combined	459

WHITE FEMALES, AGE 15–19	PER 100,000
1. Motor vehicle accidents	197
2. Suicide	52
3. Homicide	40
4. Poisonings	17
5. Leukemia	17
6. Stroke	13
7. Pneumonia	13
8. Congenital circulatory defects	11
9. Brain cancer	9
10. Drownings	8
All other causes combined	223

BLACK MALES, AGE 15–19	PER 100,000
1. Homicide	1,038
2. Motor vehicle accidents	422
3. Drownings	185
4. Suicide	123
5. Poisonings	80
6. Accidents with firearms	65
7. Accidents involving machines (excluding cars)	41
8. Pneumonia	27
9. Stroke	25
10. Fire	22
All other causes combined	813

BLACK FEMALES, AGE 15–19	PER 100,000
1. Homicide	247
2. Motor vehicle accidents	105
3. Complications of pregnancy and abortions	38
4. Poisonings	38
5. Suicide	37
6. Pneumonia	24
7. Stroke	21
8. Drownings	16
9. Fire	15
10. Rheumatic heart disease	15
All other causes combined	504

THE LONGEVITY FACTOR

WHITE MALES, AGE 20-24	PER 100,000
1. Motor vehicle accidents	581
2. Suicide	250
3. Homicide	164
4. Poisonings	69
5. Accidents involving machines (excluding cars)	64
6. Drownings	53
7. Falls	29
8. Accidents involving aircraft	28
9. Accidents with firearms	25
10. Fires	22
All other causes combined	556

WHITE FEMALES, AGE 20-24	PER 100,000
1. Motor vehicle accidents	139
2. Suicide	77
3. Homicide	45
4. Stroke	20
5. Poisonings	17
6. Leukemia	15
7. Pneumonia	15
8. Diabetes mellitus	11
9. Breast cancer	10
10. Hodgkin's disease	10
All other causes combined	291

BLACK MALES, AGE 20-24	PER 100,000
1. Homicide	1,596
2. Motor vehicle accidents	521
3. Suicide	216
4. Drownings	140
5. Poisonings	138
6. Accidents with firearms	64
7. Cirrhosis of the liver	58
8. Pneumonia	52
9. Accidents involving machines (excluding cars)	48
10. Stroke	47
Arteriosclerotic heart disease	47
All other causes combined	1,286

BLACK FEMALES, AGE 20-24	PER 100,000
1. Homicide	313
2. Motor vehicle accidents	112
3. Poisonings	51
4. Suicide	48
5. Stroke	47
6. Complications of pregnancy and abortions	45
7. Cirrhosis of the liver	38
8. Pneumonia	31
9. Arteriosclerotic heart disease	19
10. Rheumatic heart disease	19
All other causes combined	739

THE POSTPONABLE DISEASES

WHITE MALES, AGE 25–29 PER 100,000

1. Motor vehicle accidents 403
2. Suicide 240
3. Homicide 163
4. Arteriosclerotic heart disease 71
5. Accidents involving machines (excluding cars) 62
6. Poisonings 52
7. Cirrhosis of the liver 38
8. Drownings 36
9. Accidents involving aircraft 35
10. Stroke 28
All other causes combined 633

WHITE FEMALES, AGE 25–29 PER 100,000

1. Motor vehicle accidents 103
2. Suicide 91
3. Homicide 66
4. Breast cancer 38
5. Stroke 31
6. Arteriosclerotic heart disease 19
7. Cirrhosis of the liver 19
8. Diabetes mellitus 18
9. Pneumonia 18
10. Leukemia 17
All other causes combined 380

BLACK MALES, AGE 25–29 PER 100,000

1. Homicide 1,617
2. Motor vehicle accidents 472
3. Suicide 223
4. Cirrhosis of the liver 215
5. Arteriosclerotic heart disease 159
6. Poisonings 140
7. Stroke 102
8. Drownings 101
9. Pneumonia 97
10. Alcoholism 85
All other causes combined 1,687

BLACK FEMALES, AGE 25–29 PER 100,000

1. Homicide 300
2. Cirrhosis of the liver 122
3. Motor vehicle accidents 106
4. Stroke 96
5. Arteriosclerotic heart disease 76
6. Suicide 54
7. Pneumonia 51
8. Breast cancer 49
9. Complications of pregnancy and abortions 45
10. Poisonings 44
All other causes combined 1,006

THE LONGEVITY FACTOR

WHITE MALES, AGE 30-34	PER 100,000
1. Motor vehicle accidents	325
2. Arteriosclerotic heart disease	254
3. Suicide	244
4. Homicide	159
5. Cirrhosis of the liver	98
6. Accidents involving machines (excluding cars)	63
7. Stroke	56
8. Lung cancer	46
9. Poisonings	38
10. Accidents involving aircraft	37
All other causes combined	828

WHITE FEMALES, AGE 30-34	PER 100,000
1. Suicide	105
2. Breast cancer	97
3. Motor vehicle accidents	90
4. Stroke	60
5. Arteriosclerotic heart disease	54
6. Cirrhosis of the liver	49
7. Homicide	46
8. Cancer of the cervix	29
9. Lung cancer	24
10. Pneumonia	24
All other causes combined	582

BLACK MALES, AGE 30-34	PER 100,000
1. Homicide	1,501
2. Cirrhosis of the liver	448
3. Motor vehicle accidents	431
4. Arteriosclerotic heart disease	415
5. Stroke	197
6. Suicide	184
7. Pneumonia	177
8. Alcoholism	152
9. Poisonings	109
10. Drownings	96
All other causes combined	2,256

BLACK FEMALES, AGE 30-34	PER 100,000
1. Homicide	288
2. Cirrhosis of the liver	241
3. Arteriosclerotic heart disease	200
4. Stroke	187
5. Breast cancer	136
6. Motor vehicle accidents	104
7. Cancer of the cervix	97
8. Pneumonia	82
9. Alcoholism	55
10. Hypertensive heart disease	47
All other causes combined	1,455

THE POSTPONABLE DISEASES

WHITE MALES, AGE 35-39	PER 100,000	WHITE FEMALES, AGE 35-39	PER 100,000
1. Arteriosclerotic heart disease	723	1. Breast cancer	186
2. Motor vehicle accidents	290	2. Arteriosclerotic heart disease	136
3. Suicide	250	3. Suicide	125
4. Cirrhosis of the liver	200	4. Stroke	108
5. Homicide	148	5. Cirrhosis of the liver	101
6. Lung cancer	141	6. Motor vehicle accidents	91
7. Stroke	106	7. Lung cancer	66
8. Accidents involving machines (excluding cars)	63	8. Cancer of the ovary	51
9. Pneumonia	49	9. Cancer of the cervix	49
10. Cancer of the large intestine and rectum	44	10. Cancer of the large intestine and rectum	46
All other causes combined	1,167	All other causes combined	830

BLACK MALES, AGE 35-39	PER 100,000	BLACK FEMALES, AGE 35-39	PER 100,000
1. Homicide	1,340	1. Arteriosclerotic heart disease	490
2. Arteriosclerotic heart disease	977	2. Stroke	358
3. Cirrhosis of the liver	651	3. Cirrhosis of the liver	351
4. Motor vehicle accidents	422	4. Homicide	259
5. Stroke	384	5. Breast cancer	251
6. Lung cancer	254	6. Cancer of the cervix	148
7. Pneumonia	249	7. Pneumonia	111
8. Alcoholism	205	8. Motor vehicle accidents	99
9. Suicide	153	9. Alcoholism	88
10. Hypertensive heart disease	102	10. Lung cancer	82
All other causes combined	3,127	All other causes combined	2,071

THE LONGEVITY FACTOR

WHITE MALES, AGE 40–44	PER 100,000
1. Arteriosclerotic heart disease	1,629
2. Lung cancer	348
3. Cirrhosis of the liver	343
4. Motor vehicle accidents	275
5. Suicide	260
6. Stroke	178
7. Homicide	128
8. Cancer of the large intestine and rectum	86
9. Pneumonia	75
10. Accidents involving machines (excluding cars)	63
All other causes combined	1,750

WHITE FEMALES, AGE 40–44	PER 100,000
1. Breast cancer	342
2. Arteriosclerotic heart disease	308
3. Stroke	174
4. Cirrhosis of the liver	170
5. Lung cancer	149
6. Suicide	143
7. Cancer of the ovary	101
8. Motor vehicle accidents	93
9. Cancer of the large intestine and rectum	87
10. Cancer of the cervix	70
All other causes combined	1,215

BLACK MALES, AGE 40–44	PER 100,000
1. Arteriosclerotic heart disease	2,034
2. Homicide	1,110
3. Cirrhosis of the liver	834
4. Stroke	677
5. Lung cancer	607
6. Motor vehicle accidents	393
7. Pneumonia	322
8. Alcoholism	266
9. Hypertensive heart disease	154
10. Falls	145
All other causes combined	4,230

BLACK FEMALES, AGE 40–44	PER 100,000
1. Arteriosclerotic heart disease	1,061
2. Stroke	597
3. Cirrhosis of the liver	468
4. Breast cancer	404
5. Homicide	196
6. Lung cancer	194
7. Cancer of the cervix	182
8. Pneumonia	143
9. Hypertensive heart disease	128
10. Nephritis and nephrosis	104
All other causes combined	2,867

THE POSTPONABLE DISEASES

WHITE MALES, AGE 45–49	PER 100,000
1. Arteriosclerotic heart disease	2,973
2. Lung cancer	681
3. Cirrhosis of the liver	471
4. Stroke	299
5. Suicide	281
6. Motor vehicle accidents	260
7. Cancer of the large intestine and rectum	172
8. Pneumonia	113
9. Homicide	109
10. Bronchitis and emphysema	88
All other causes combined	2,158

WHITE FEMALES, AGE 45–49	PER 100,000
1. Arteriosclerotic heart disease	624
2. Breast cancer	518
3. Stroke	268
4. Lung cancer	249
5. Cirrhosis of the liver	232
6. Cancer of the ovary	162
7. Cancer of the large intestine and rectum	161
8. Suicide	145
9. Motor vehicle accidents	92
10. Cancer of the cervix	90
All other causes combined	1,767

BLACK MALES, AGE 45–49	PER 100,000
1. Arteriosclerotic heart disease	3,476
2. Lung cancer	1,183
3. Stroke	1,029
4. Homicide	987
5. Cirrhosis of the liver	919
6. Pneumonia	416
7. Motor vehicle accidents	391
8. Alcoholism	297
9. Cancer of the esophagus	255
10. Hypertensive heart disease	223
All other causes combined	5,606

BLACK FEMALES, AGE 45–49	PER 100,000
1. Arteriosclerotic heart disease	1,834
2. Stroke	893
3. Breast cancer	584
4. Cirrhosis of the liver	486
5. Lung cancer	311
6. Cancer of the cervix	217
7. Hypertensive heart disease	196
8. Pneumonia	180
9. Cancer of the large intestine and rectum	172
10. Homicide	162
All other causes combined	3,865

THE LONGEVITY FACTOR

WHITE MALES, AGE 50-54	PER 100,000
1. Arteriosclerotic heart disease	5,001
2. Lung cancer	1,188
3. Cirrhosis of the liver	580
4. Stroke	541
5. Cancer of the large intestine and rectum	314
6. Suicide	301
7. Motor vehicle accidents	248
8. Bronchitis and emphysema	198
9. Pneumonia	191
10. Rheumatic heart disease	123
All other causes combined	4,038

WHITE FEMALES, AGE 50-54	PER 100,000
1. Arteriosclerotic heart disease	1,260
2. Breast cancer	684
3. Stroke	422
4. Lung cancer	386
5. Cirrhosis of the liver	284
6. Cancer of the large intestine and rectum	277
7. Cancer of the ovary	227
8. Suicide	131
9. Rheumatic heart disease	111
10. Cancer of the cervix	103
All other causes combined	2,604

BLACK MALES, AGE 50-54	PER 100,000
1. Arteriosclerotic heart disease	5,332
2. Lung cancer	1,893
3. Stroke	1,583
4. Cirrhosis of the liver	878
5. Homicide	806
6. Pneumonia	533
7. Motor vehicle accidents	410
8. Cancer of the esophagus	393
9. Hypertensive heart disease	299
10. Cancer of the stomach	293
All other causes combined	7,803

BLACK FEMALES, AGE 50-54	PER 100,000
1. Arteriosclerotic heart disease	3,042
2. Stroke	1,348
3. Breast cancer	703
4. Cirrhosis of the liver	458
5. Lung cancer	421
6. Cancer of the large intestine and rectum	316
7. Hypertensive heart disease	297
8. Cancer of the cervix	272
9. Pneumonia	207
10. Nephritis and nephrosis	185
All other causes combined	5,155

THE POSTPONABLE DISEASES

WHITE MALES, AGE 55–59	PER 100,000
1. Arteriosclerotic heart disease	7,809
2. Lung cancer	1,888
3. Stroke	979
4. Cirrhosis of the liver	667
5. Cancer of the large intestine and rectum	530
6. Bronchitis and emphysema	411
7. Pneumonia	312
8. Suicide	307
9. Motor vehicle accidents	258
10. Cancer of the stomach	192
All other causes combined	6,085

WHITE FEMALES, AGE 55–59	PER 100,000
1. Arteriosclerotic heart disease	2,406
2. Breast cancer	807
3. Stroke	699
4. Lung cancer	517
5. Cancer of the large intestine and rectum	434
6. Cirrhosis of the liver	311
7. Cancer of the ovary	284
8. Rheumatic heart disease	166
9. Pneumonia	148
10. Bronchitis and emphysema	148
All other causes combined	3,697

BLACK MALES, AGE 55–59	PER 100,000
1. Arteriosclerotic heart disease	7,608
2. Lung cancer	2,437
3. Stroke	2,400
4. Cirrhosis of the liver	783
5. Pneumonia	683
6. Homicide	612
7. Cancer of the prostate	499
8. Cancer of the large intestine and rectum	487
9. Cancer of the esophagus	443
10. Cancer of the stomach	434
All other causes combined	10,176

BLACK FEMALES, AGE 55–59	PER 100,000
1. Arteriosclerotic heart disease	4,697
2. Stroke	2,007
3. Breast cancer	730
4. Cancer of the large intestine and rectum	491
5. Lung cancer	487
6. Cirrhosis of the liver	402
7. Hypertensive heart disease	384
8. Cancer of the cervix	308
9. Pneumonia	258
10. Nephritis and nephrosis	246
All other causes combined	6,683

THE LONGEVITY FACTOR

WHITE MALES, AGE 60-64	PER 100,000
1. Arteriosclerotic heart disease	11,273
2. Lung cancer	2,561
3. Stroke	1,775
4. Cancer of the large intestine and rectum	814
5. Bronchitis and emphysema	736
6. Cirrhosis of the liver	693
7. Pneumonia	483
8. Cancer of the prostate	422
9. Suicide	289
10. Diseases of the arteries	284
All other causes combined	8,517

WHITE FEMALES, AGE 60-64	PER 100,000
1. Arteriosclerotic heart disease	4,307
2. Stroke	1,241
3. Breast cancer	859
4. Cancer of the large intestine and rectum	631
5. Lung cancer	501
6. Cancer of the ovary	319
7. Cirrhosis of the liver	290
8. Pneumonia	231
9. Rheumatic heart disease	227
10. Bronchitis and emphysema	208
All other causes combined	5,156

BLACK MALES, AGE 60-64	PER 100,000
1. Arteriosclerotic heart disease	10,138
2. Stroke	3,514
3. Lung cancer	2,709
4. Cancer of the prostate	984
5. Pneumonia	856
6. Cancer of the large intestine and rectum	716
7. Cirrhosis of the liver	621
8. Cancer of the stomach	594
9. Hypertensive heart disease	543
10. Homicide	461
All other causes combined	12,048

BLACK FEMALES, AGE 60-64	PER 100,000
1. Arteriosclerotic heart disease	6,782
2. Stroke	3,032
3. Breast cancer	748
4. Cancer of the large intestine and rectum	638
5. Hypertensive heart disease	512
6. Lung cancer	458
7. Pneumonia	369
8. Cancer of the cervix	309
9. Cirrhosis of the liver	276
10. Nephritis and nephrosis	273
All other causes combined	8,281

THE POSTPONABLE DISEASES

WHITE MALES, AGE 65-69	PER 100,000
1. Arteriosclerotic heart disease	15,622
2. Stroke	3,218
3. Lung cancer	2,998
4. Bronchitis and emphysema	1,152
5. Cancer of the large intestine and rectum	1,121
6. Cancer of the prostate	809
7. Pneumonia	785
8. Cirrhosis of the liver	615
9. Diseases of the arteries	519
10. Cancer of the stomach	368
All other causes combined	11,180

WHITE FEMALES, AGE 65-69	PER 100,000
1. Arteriosclerotic heart disease	7,755
2. Stroke	2,464
3. Breast cancer	921
4. Cancer of the large intestine and rectum	900
5. Diseases of the arteries	388
6. Pneumonia	383
7. Cancer of the ovary	335
8. Rheumatic heart disease	279
9. Bronchitis and emphysema	264
10. Cirrhosis of the liver	245
All other causes combined	7,430

BLACK MALES, AGE 65-69	PER 100,000
1. Arteriosclerotic heart disease	14,229
2. Stroke	5,367
3. Lung cancer	2,958
4. Cancer of the prostate	1,820
5. Pneumonia	1,165
6. Cancer of the large intestine and rectum	971
7. Hypertensive heart disease	772
8. Cancer of the stomach	753
9. Diseases of the arteries	612
10. Bronchitis and emphysema	550
All other cases combined	14,637

BLACK FEMALES, AGE 65-69	PER 100,000
1. Arteriosclerotic heart disease	11,110
2. Stroke	5,210
3. Cancer of the large intestine and rectum	946
4. Breast cancer	826
5. Hypertensive heart disease	800
6. Diseases of the arteries	654
7. Pneumonia	653
8. Lung cancer	465
9. Cancer of the stomach	404
10. Cancer of the uterus	359
All other causes combined	11,220

THE LONGEVITY FACTOR

WHITE MALES, AGE 70–74	PER 100,000
1. Arteriosclerotic heart disease	21,374
2. Stroke	5,583
3. Lung cancer	3,176
4. Bronchitis and emphysema	1,552
5. Cancer of the large intestine and rectum	1,464
6. Pneumonia	1,431
7. Cancer of the prostate	1,400
8. Diseases of the arteries	953
9. Cancer of the stomach	510
10. Cancer of the bladder	479
All other causes combined	14,438

WHITE FEMALES, AGE 70–74	PER 100,000
1. Arteriosclerotic heart disease	13,666
2. Stroke	5,079
3. Cancer of the large intestine and rectum	1,232
4. Breast cancer	1,018
5. Diseases of the arteries	853
6. Pneumonia	777
7. Lung cancer	564
8. Hypertensive heart disease	394
9. Cancer of the ovary	347
10. Bronchitis and emphysema	314
All other causes combined	9,909

BLACK MALES, AGE 70–74	PER 100,000
1. Arteriosclerotic heart disease	18,323
2. Stroke	7,382
3. Lung cancer	2,834
4. Cancer of the prostate	2,671
5. Pneumonia	1,677
6. Cancer of the large intestine and rectum	1,282
7. Diseases of the arteries	960
8. Hypertensive heart disease	941
9. Cancer of the stomach	830
10. Bronchitis and emphysema	607
All other causes combined	17,064

BLACK FEMALES, AGE 70–74	PER 100,000
1. Arteriosclerotic heart disease	15,157
2. Stroke	7,485
3. Cancer of the large intestine and rectum	1,133
4. Diseases of the arteries	1,082
5. Hypertensive heart disease	1,016
6. Pneumonia	936
7. Breast cancer	812
8. Cancer of the stomach	492
9. Lung cancer	480
10. Nephritis and nephrosis	410
All other causes combined	13,462

PART II

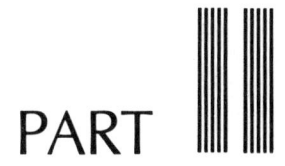

In the section that follows, you will find the chronicles of nine people who have taken hard looks at their health prospects, and made up their minds to change their ways and add years to their lives. Some of them used various types of profiling to help; others now wish they had been able to. There are winners and losers here. Not all the names are real; some were changed to preserve privacy. These stories may help you to make a few changes of your own.

5
AGE 40—
TIME TO GROW UP:
Donald Hanson, Alcoholic

Donald Hanson has a job he likes and is good at; he makes $25,000 a year as a welfare administrator in a sizable Texas city. He is 43 years old but looks younger, with boyish brown eyes and curly brown hair. He has a ready laugh.

"I'm not just one more alcoholic," he says sardonically. "I've got family tradition behind me.

"My father was a happy alcoholic. He would play the piano for hours, and sing.

"But my grandfather, he was a mean alcoholic. Once, when my father was 11 years old, my grandfather held him up by the hair and smashed him in the face with his fist, breaking his nose. My grandmother left the old man after that."

Hanson himself followed yet a different pattern. He became what is called a periodic drinker. He would stay sober for weeks, but tension would be building up inside him; when it reached a certain point he would go off by himself and drink steadily for two or three days, disappearing into alcohol.

The son of a building contractor, Don spent his childhood in St. Paul, Minnesota, where he learned about drinking at an early age. "From the beginning my parents partied a lot, both of them. There were always people dropping in, having drinks," he recalls. "My father liked to drink and play that piano. He was a super kind of person, very decent, very kind."

When the parties were over, Don as a little boy rounded up the empty beer bottles. "You should have seen my room: racks and racks of beer bottles, like a supermarket. Then I'd take 'em out—sell 'em, get good money for 'em.

"It was a pretty stable life, actually. On a Sunday morning I could go for Swedish pancakes to my Grandma Hanson's house across the street, or else go wake my Irish grandfather up the hill—he was about 80, and he made sour-dough pancakes. Relatives and neighbors were always around."

It was at one of the family parties that Don, 18 years old and about to enter the army, got drunk for the first time. He became the object of much affectionate teasing.

It was decided that someone had better walk him around the block. "It was a big long block, with a lot of trees," he recalls. "On the way I got to feeling sick to my stomach, and I had to stop and vomit. I remember the people with me laughing and giggling.

"Well, I got back home again and went into the bathroom and looked at myself in the mirror, and that's when I realized my two front teeth were missing. You see, they'd been knocked out a few years before in a football game, and I had this bridge that I wore. The bridge must have popped out when I was vomiting.

"So we got out the flashlight—it was nighttime, you

know—" Hanson is laughing, his brown eyes dancing, "—and retraced our steps, and sort of rooted round, and sure enough, there was my bridge. Took it home, washed it off, put it back in my mouth, and I was as good as new.

"Oh, everyone thought that was just great. I remember everyone saying how cute that was."

His tone is carefree. He isn't blaming anyone. Yet he clearly remembers that he didn't enjoy his first drunk. Looking back on that milestone of his life, destined to be repeated so often in the years to come, he says thoughtfully, "You know, drinking never did make me happy. My mother, when she drank, would get very obnoxious. I'm like her in that—didn't want to be, but I am. It's my opinion that I'm allergic to alcohol, and have been from the beginning."

During the next few years drinking played only a small part in Don's life. His term in the army over, his major problem was school. Though obviously bright, he had always had trouble studying. In all, he attended seven different colleges and flunked out of six of them; at the seventh, he finally gave up without a degree. For several years he "sort of drifted around." In 1959 he married LaVerne Hickey, a schoolteacher, and settled down in east Texas.

Then, unexpectedly, he was offered a job at a center for retarded children, took it, and found that he loved the work. His career was under way.

Since then Hanson has worked with prison inmates; with the chronic indigent; with battered and neglected children; with juvenile delinquents; and, most recently, in welfare. He is good at what he does—he has had to be, to make up for his poor academic credentials and his drinking.

During the 1960s the drinking began leading to incidents. Heading home from a party one night in 1963, he drove his car across a highway divider, flattening his tires in the process; then, feeling shaken, he pulled off the road. Someone in a nearby house witnessed what happened and called the police. Hanson spent the rest of the night in jail.

Not long afterward Hanson lost his job at the retarded children's center, following a policy fight with an elected official. He worked for a season as a minor league baseball umpire, but when that ran out, so did his money. Within a year he found himself on welfare and legally bankrupt, his home taken from him in a mortgage foreclosure. It was during this same period that his father died suddenly, aged 56, of a heart attack.

These events weighed hard on Hanson, and more and more he tried to dispel the strain by drinking. He began suffering memory blackouts, sometimes waking up in a strange room with no idea of how he'd gotten there.

Luck returned: once again he found a job in his chosen field. But his alcohol consumption continued to rise, and it wasn't long before he was in trouble again, this time in the form of an affair with a young woman in his new office. This began near Christmas 1967, and did not last long—the emotional involvement, the guilt, he says, were more than he could handle. He remembers going out drinking with her one night, then almost driving his car through a store window on the way home. "I don't know. Everything was suddenly too much for me. I decided to quit drinking."

In hindsight, the decision was a superficial one—"like going swimming on January first; I wanted to see if I could do it." Nevertheless, he managed to last eighteen months without liquor. Then, reassured, he began drinking again.

Don's drinking had always happened in response to the stresses in his life; the early 1970s provided him with plenty of these. Relations with his wife and two sons had been deteriorating for several years, largely because of his drinking. Now, suddenly, his working life, so important to him,

AGE 40—TIME TO GROW UP

was thrown into turmoil as scandals hit the welfare department of his county. The trouble began in 1970 and lasted off and on through 1975, leading to a grand jury investigation, many firings, and countless newspaper headlines. "Our own little Watergate," he explains drily. Some of the administrators he worked closely with, men he admired and respected, came under attack, and two of them suffered coronaries—a result of the stress they were under, in Don's opinion. In 1974 Don's own position was threatened.

At the height of the investigation, Don came home one day feeling depressed. It was four o'clock, a time when he was usually still at work. He opened his front door and headed down the hall. "I should have known better, I guess. Anyway, this was when I discovered my wife was involved with another man."

Hanson felt crushed by the discovery, *"very,* very bitter." He began seeing a psychotherapist. In fact, during this period of marital troubles plus the grand jury pressures, he saw several therapists at various times. None of them helped much—perhaps because he never quite leveled with them about his drinking. His wife embarked on therapy too; the two compared notes during amiable interludes.

And of course Don drank, more heavily than ever. "I got so I wouldn't stay in the community, I'd drive down to Galveston instead, where my brother lived. Usually I'd drink with him and his beatnik friends. These people were drunk half the time.

"Or I'd go into a bar by myself and drink alone." He is thoughtful a moment. He says, "You know what a bar makes me think of? A church. Seriously. You go in. You're recognized. It's kind of dark in there. You can sit by yourself and have personal fantasies. It's kind of a place to hide. A quiet place.

"Of course, after I'd been there drinking a while, it might not be all that quiet. I can get very unpleasant when I'm drunk. Liquor is supposed to make you feel good. You know what used to make *me* feel good? Throwing up—vomiting. There'd be that terrible pain in the head, and all that mess and obnoxiousness. But afterward I'd sort of be at peace. The emotions I had been dealing with would be gone for a while, the tensions would disappear."

Through this period Hanson, beneath the surface, was feeling deeply depressed—and not a little paranoid as well, at moments. "For some reason I became convinced the law was after me," he says. "I was down in Galveston with my brother one night, drinking. It got to be very late. I suppose we were making a lot of noise. Anyway, there came a pounding on the door, a voice said, 'It's the police.' Evidently a neighbor had complained. But at the moment all I could think of was the police back home. I thought, *The police chief is trying to set me up; he planned this.* I was just very, very scared."

In childhood Don had once been diagnosed as having a possible heart murmur. Now, as his fortieth birthday approached, he began worrying about his health. For a couple of years he had not felt well physically. He suffered from chest pains and shortness of breath. He could not help thinking of his father, struck down at the age of 56, a man in seemingly excellent health.

He also found himself thinking about his mother, still alive. Since her husband's death she had been arrested twice for drunken driving.

He began wondering too about his sons, aged 16 and 12, and what kind of a model he must be for them. In a few years they would grow up and leave home.

At work, the scandals and investigations had ended at last, bringing a kind of pause into Hanson's life. He looked back. He saw that for many years he had lived a life of

AGE 40—TIME TO GROW UP

highs and lows, passing from peak to trough to peak again. A feeling of weariness took possession of him. He wasn't just tired; he was tired of being tired. "In short, a lot came together for me in 1975. A lot."

This time there was nothing impulsive about his decision. He thought it over dispassionately for several weeks. Then he stopped drinking.

Don remembers not only the first drink he ever had, but also the last, at an office party. He had spent the day out of town on business; when he finally arrived back, about seven in the evening, the party was in full swing. "Just about everybody was drunk by then," he remembers wryly, "literally. The chief probation officer was bombed out of his mind—practically falling on the floor."

Don had stopped smoking a week earlier, by way of a church program. At the party he had three drinks, and even smoked a few cigarettes. He did not become intoxicated, and he has not had a drink or a cigarette since.

Hanson stopped drinking on his own, without guidance from anyone. A week after quitting, however, he went to see a doctor—he wanted to investigate that heart murmur—and in the course of the visit was invited to fill out a health profile questionnaire. He complied, automatically expecting the worst. But the results, when they came, surprised and reassured him. Forty-one-year-old Donald Hanson, who was now both an ex-drinker and ex-smoker, was told he was running the health risks of the average white male of 42. "And I *could* be 38, if I would do thus and so and thus and so. That didn't sound like I was so badly off."

Not as badly off as he was feeling. At the time he saw the doctor, he was still suffering sharp chest pains, numbness in the arms, and emphysema-like respiratory symptoms.

It is difficult enough to conquer a single addictive habit,

but Hanson attacked two at once: he stopped drinking and smoking simultaneously. What was it like the first few days, that first month, without the alcohol and nicotine that had raggedly sustained him for so many years? Hanson is not particularly anxious to remember. "There were tough times all right," is about as far as he likes to go. "I purposely haven't attempted to analyze them. What I did was necessary, that I know."

He remembers sleeping a lot. "I'd sleep all morning Saturday morning. In effect, I was catching up on two or three years of exhaustion." He also ate, and before long weighed 232 pounds.

Very gradually he began, as he puts it, getting his house in order. "Another ex-drinker I know went through the same business: during his first year he cleaned out every closet in his house. Spent a solid year cleaning closets!" Don is laughing. "Well," he continues, "I was like him. I just began sorting things out. By now I guess I've sorted out everything there *is* in my life—caught up on all the things I'd been neglecting over the years. There were a lot of them."

Soon after his visit to the doctor, Don found, and joined, an Alcoholics Anonymous chapter in town which meets each Tuesday. He says that his particular group is somewhat unusual—"all professional people—doctors, attorneys, a few psychiatrists, people with special positions in town, making it difficult for them to reveal a drinking problem. From the very beginning I liked them; I just fit."

One of the ways AA helped him was by giving him something to do— "a way to fill the void," as he puts it—that not drinking created in his life. In addition, through his new friends in AA he became involved in a professional society consisting chiefly of lawyers and psychologists; Don is currently vice president of this group, and recently ran a workshop on the use of behavioral sciences in the judicial process.

Soon after joining AA, Don says he began having strange experiences, of a type he'd already heard about from a fellow AA member, who described them, quite simply, as miracles. Don says, "I sort of discounted what he said. But then these coincidences began happening to me. Everything from getting the new job I wanted, to relationships with people. I'd be worried about a problem during the day, and I'd come home at night and watch educational TV, and there'd be a show about it. When I was concerned about something else, I'd meet the guy the next day and solve that problem. Eventually I just got accustomed to this sort of thing. Understand, these were the kinds of problems I used to raise hell about, fight battles over. I don't know. Maybe I seek things now that I didn't seek before.

"Another thing about alcoholics: they stop dreaming, did you know that? Now I dream regularly again."

Physically he feels good these days, and he is taking steps to feel better. His doctor has told him he definitely has no heart murmur, so he has applied for admission to an exercise program administered by a local college. "Running and swimming chiefly," he says. "It's for the heart and lungs, of course, but also to increase your energy level. The program's very systematic: they weigh you under water, all that kind of thing. I've always been attracted by very objective data. It's one of the things I like about health profiling."

Hanson asserts that the happiest period in his life has been the two years since he quit drinking and smoking. "The happiest since I was 18 years old," he says. "Eighteen to 40: that's a long time not to have a real handle on things." He pauses, his pleasant face serious. "You narrow down to the important things. My marriage—I was worried about it—is working out. My job's going well. But what matters the most is how I feel about myself. I feel that I'm mature now. I feel I'm in control."

Once in a while he wonders what would happen if he got involved again in a major crisis, such as the grand jury investigation. And he looks back and remembers. "I used to get these tremendous bursts of energy. You know, between all the pressures and the alcohol. And when I decided to stop drinking, I remember honestly wondering, *Now what am I going to do without the things that charge me up?* Like, *Where's my next grand jury investigation?* I felt like a punchdrunk fighter: someone'd ring the bell, and I'd come out and start going like this." He weaves his clenched fists in front of him, laughing.

The laughter fades. "There used to be big highs in my life. Not now." He says quietly, "I'm just very happy to be sane."

* * *

Health profiling has become a part of Don's annual physical examination, and to study his printouts is to follow the ups and downs of a by now veteran habit changer—his progress and, sometimes, the complications that progress produces.

His first profile is dated October 15, 1975, just a couple of weeks after he stopped drinking and smoking. His chronological age at the time was 41. His risk age was 42, but he was informed he could reduce it four years, mainly by getting more exercise and by seeking help for the depressed moods he had been suffering. His blood pressure was also a shade above average, and he was 18 percent overweight, matters at least to think about.

Fifteen months later he filled out his second questionnaire. Adjusted now to living without alcohol or cigarettes, he no longer felt depressed, so his ten-year risk for suicide had dropped by more than half. He'd also begun exercising—not a lot, but the equivalent of a one-mile walk four times a week: this alone took 1.7 years off his risk age. He'd even begun fastening his seat belt more often.

But closely linked to his gains came losses, side effects, one might call them, of Hanson's well-intended self-therapy. Like many ex-smokers, he was eating too much: he was now 36 percent overweight and his blood level of triglycerides had nearly doubled. In addition, his diastolic blood pressure was up to 94, compared with 88 fifteen months earlier. This change may well have been related to overeating; blood pressure tends to increase with weight.

The result was that in January 1977 Don's medical age was two years older than his actual age, compared with a difference of only one year in October 1975. Discouraging? Not necessarily, the message was so clear. What Don had to do now was to get control of his weight, preferably through both diet and exercise.

Since that time he has made steady progress. By January 1978, when he returned for his third health profile, his blood pressure was down to 130/90; and his weight, too, appeared to have turned around: he had lost 8 pounds, compared with a gain of 34 the year before.

But what really pleased Don was the way these modest changes, along with a few others, affected his overall risk, carrying him across a kind of magic threshold. At 43 years of age, his printout informed him, he suddenly had the health prospects of a man of 42.

One final speculation: If Don had made none of these changes, had never stirred himself to take that first giant step of dropping alcohol and tobacco from his life, what would his risks be today? The answer is easily obtainable; just take his 1975 questionnaire, add to it 3 years of age, 40 or more drinks per week, and 1½ packs of cigarettes per day, and submit it to a computer. What's the result? A health profile in which cirrhosis of the liver heads the list of risks, with grossly elevated ratings as well for heart disease, motor vehicle accidents, suicide, lung cancer, homicide, and pneumonia. If Hanson still drank today, his risk of auto accident death would be almost 10 times that of a nondrinker—of cirrhosis, 100 times. And his risk age would be 51—rather than the 42 it actually is, two and a half years since he stopped drinking and smoking.

Here is Hanson's most recent profile, the one he likes best:

HEALTH RISK PROFILE

Donald Hanson, age 43, white.

Age in terms of present health, 42.

Achievable health age, 40.

An average white man your age has 5,135 chances per 100,000 of dying in the next ten years; your risks are 9% less than average. You can, however, reduce these risks by 27%.

FACTORS OFFERING THE GREATEST REDUCTION IN RISK:	THE NUMBER OF YEARS TO BE GAINED BY ALTERING THOSE FACTORS:
Weight	.9 year
Blood pressure	.3 year
Smoking (remaining stopped)	.2 year
Cholesterol	.1 year
Exercise	.1 year
Other factors	.4 year
Total	2.0 years

AGE 40—TIME TO GROW UP

Your risks of death within the next ten years in descending importance:

1. ARTERIOSCLEROTIC HEART DISEASE (heart attack)

AVERAGE RISK	1,629 ●●●●●●●●●●
YOUR CURRENT RISK	1,580 ●●●●●●●●●●
YOUR ACHIEVABLE RISK	635 ●●●●

INDICATORS OF RISK	RISK RATING	WAYS TO REDUCE RISK	RISK RATING
Blood pressure: current, 130/90 average of current and previous, 134/89	.9	Blood pressure 120/80 or less	.6
Current cholesterol 193	.7	Cholesterol 180 or lower	.6
Diabetes—none	1.0		
Exercise—moderate	.6	Exercise—vigorous	.5
Family history of early heart deaths—one parent	1.2		
Former smoker	.7	Remain stopped	.5
Weight—31% overweight	1.3	Reduce to average	1.0
History of abnormal electrocardiogram— none	1.0		
Triglycerides: current, 192 average of current and previous, 200	1.2	Reduce to 151 or less	1.1

Excessive stress may increase risk. Exact risk factor not yet available.

2. LUNG CANCER

AVERAGE RISK	348 ●●●●●●●●●●
YOUR CURRENT RISK	278 ●●●●●●●●
YOUR ACHIEVABLE RISK	278 ●●●●●●●●

THE LONGEVITY FACTOR

INDICATORS OF RISK	RISK RATING	WAYS TO REDUCE RISK	RISK RATING
Former smoker	.8	Remain stopped	.8
		Remain stopped 7 years	.2

3. SUICIDE

AVERAGE RISK	260 ●●●●●●●●●●
YOUR CURRENT RISK	260 ●●●●●●●●●●
YOUR ACHIEVABLE RISK	260 ●●●●●●●●●●

INDICATORS OF RISK	RISK RATING	WAYS TO REDUCE RISK	RISK RATING
Depression—none	1.0		
Family history of suicide—none	1.0		
Former drinker	1.0		

4. MOTOR VEHICLE ACCIDENTS

AVERAGE RISK	275 ●●●●●●●●●●
YOUR CURRENT RISK	193 ●●●●●●●
YOUR ACHIEVABLE RISK	165 ●●●●●●

INDICATORS OF RISK	RISK RATING	WAYS TO REDUCE RISK	RISK RATING
Former drinker	.5		
Mileage—20,000 yearly as driver or passenger	1.2		
Seat belt use—10% to 24% of time	1.0	Use seat belts always	.8

5. HOMICIDE

AVERAGE RISK	128 ●●●●●●●●●●
YOUR CURRENT RISK	128 ●●●●●●●●●●
YOUR ACHIEVABLE RISK	128 ●●●●●●●●●●

AGE 40—TIME TO GROW UP

INDICATORS OF RISK	RISK RATING	WAYS TO REDUCE RISK	RISK RATING
No arrests for violence	1.0		
Does not carry weapon	1.0		
Former drinker	1.0		

6. STROKE

AVERAGE RISK	178 ••••••••••	
YOUR CURRENT RISK	112 ••••••	
YOUR ACHIEVABLE RISK	75 ••••	

INDICATORS OF RISK	RISK RATING	WAYS TO REDUCE RISK	RISK RATING
Blood pressure—average of current and previous, 134/89	.9	Blood pressure 120/80 or less	.6
Current cholesterol 193	.7		
Diabetes—none	1.0		
Former smoker	1.0		
History of abnormal electrocardiogram—none	1.0		

7. CANCER OF THE LARGE INTESTINE AND RECTUM

AVERAGE RISK	86 ••••••••••
YOUR CURRENT RISK	86 ••••••••••
YOUR ACHIEVABLE RISK	86 ••••••••••

INDICATORS OF RISK	RISK RATING	WAYS TO REDUCE RISK	RISK RATING
Intestinal polyps—none	1.0		
Rectal bleeding—none	1.0		
Ulcerative colitis—none	1.0		

THE LONGEVITY FACTOR

8. PNEUMONIA

AVERAGE RISK	75 ●●●●●●●●●●
YOUR CURRENT RISK	75 ●●●●●●●●●●
YOUR ACHIEVABLE RISK	75 ●●●●●●●●●●

INDICATORS OF RISK	RISK RATING	WAYS TO REDUCE RISK	RISK RATING
Former drinker	1.0		
No history of bacterial pneumonia	1.0		
No history of emphysema	1.0		
Former smoker	1.0		

9. CIRRHOSIS OF THE LIVER

AVERAGE RISK	343 ●●●●●●●●●●
YOUR CURRENT RISK	69 ●●
YOUR ACHIEVABLE RISK	69 ●●

INDICATORS OF RISK	RISK RATING	WAYS TO REDUCE RISK	RISK RATING
Former drinker	.2		
Liver function test normal	1.0		

10. ACCIDENTS INVOLVING MACHINES (excluding cars)

AVERAGE RISK	63 ●●●●●●●●●●
YOUR CURRENT RISK	63 ●●●●●●●●●●
YOUR ACHIEVABLE RISK	63 ●●●●●●●●●●

No risk indicators have been established for this cause of death.

AGE 40—TIME TO GROW UP

OTHER

Your risk of death from all other causes in the next ten years totals 1,750 out of 100,000.

6
QUITTING WHILE YOU'RE AHEAD:
Laura Blake, Smoker

Barely 19 years old, Laura Blake has beautiful eyes and skin, and a slim, straight-backed seriousness of manner. She wears a shoulder-length mane of gleaming brown hair, washed every day. Answering questions reflectively, she occasionally reaches back and winds her hair close around her head. Her sweater is fine, thin cashmere, clinging to her slim breasts, and worn above Calvin Klein jeans. She looks like a rather rich, confident girl, which she is, the second daughter of a New York financier and real estate operator. She was born in a well-to-do Long Island suburb, then her father moved the family out into a wealthier, more rural setting. Driving through it, one can examine the beginnings of driveways, but not many of the houses, which are discreetly set back in the countryside.

Laura looks right at you with those perfect eyes and speaks deliberately. Her diction has that upper-class urban edge known, at the eastern college where she is a freshman, as the "Long Guyland" accent.

QUITTING WHILE YOU'RE AHEAD

When did you begin smoking?
I was 13. My sister, who was 15 and smoked all the time, said, "Why don't you take a drag?" so I did, but it was a while before I started smoking regularly.

How long?
Maybe a year. When I was 14 I went to a wedding reception. I was in a bathroom with five other girls, all of us smoking. I guess we smoked most of a pack. One of the girls was trying to teach us to inhale.

It was an out-of-the-way upstairs bathroom. Everybody else was downstairs, a real big crowd. The father was a doctor, and this was his bathroom. One of the waiters told us we could use it.

Before we went downstairs we hid the pack under a towel.

For a long time I just smoked at parties or when my parents weren't around. They have an apartment in the city too, so they're not always home.

Do they smoke?
My father smokes a pipe and my mother smokes cigarettes—a lot of them. Every once in a while she'll say, "I want to quit, but I can't. If I stopped smoking, I'd start eating." But she eats anyway. My mother was always closer to my sister, and my father closer to me.

Did your high school let you smoke?
Yes. It was a day school, a private one, and we were allowed to smoke in the back parking lot. But everybody smoked in the bathrooms too. It was an accepted thing. There were no health classes or anything to discourage us. They probably wouldn't have worked anyway.

You've been smoking how long, then?
Five years.

73

When did your parents find out about it, and how did they react?

My father was always very much against cigarettes. (A pipe is not smoking, according to him.) He used to tell me that if he ever caught me smoking he would break my arm, and after I started I was so scared he would find out. One New Year's Eve we went out to our club for dinner, and me and this fellow I was seeing were in the library smoking, when my father came in to get us for dinner. We put out our cigarettes really quickly, and he didn't say anything—I wasn't sure he had noticed. But the next day (Laura smiles), I got yelled at for three hours by my mother and then three hours by my father.

After that they wouldn't let me smoke in front of them, so I smoked in my room with the door closed. But after a few months they decided that was ridiculous, and then they let me smoke in front of them.

In front of my mother didn't bother me at all, but in front of my father I felt guilty every time I took a drag. I never got used to it. When he and I went anywhere alone, I would leave my cigarettes home and not smoke.

Your father knew your sister smoked?

Yes, but I never heard of any conflict about it, though she started younger than I did. It was at my sister's twelfth birthday party that all of a sudden I saw her sitting there with a cigarette. At that time I was strongly opposed to smoking.

After you began smoking regularly, how much did you smoke?

When I was 15, a pack a day. And then Marlboro started putting more airholes in the filter so the cigarettes were weaker. After that, it was a pack and a half a day.

When did you smoke?

All the time, except early in the morning. When I was at

school, I was buying a carton a week at the least. But it was, like, ridiculous. I didn't like the whole thing, the taste in my mouth, anything. My mother gave me this $175 lighter, and I lost it a month later.

When did you first consider stopping?
One day two years ago I decided to give it up, just decided, and I made it for a day or two. But I suffered. I didn't really *want* to stop then. It was just an idea in my head.

Then last fall this girl at school told me that she had started going to Smokenders. It didn't work for her, but I asked around and found a lot of people who had graduated from it, like my gynecologist. I decided that when summer came I was going to take the course and quit.

The Smokenders meetings were at the Biltmore Hotel in New York. They cost $170 for nine meetings, but it wasn't out of my pocket, because my mother said she would pay for it. All I had to worry about was driving into the city every week.

Parking in the city is enough to make you want a cigarette, isn't it?
My father has a garage there.

What were the meetings like?
They lasted two or two and a half hours, with about fifty people. The first few meetings the room was full of smoke. The group leader talks about why you smoke—there are all kinds of reasons, hundreds of them they've figured out—and what it does to you, and they give you a lot of assignments.

Like what?
They give you a printed timetable to wrap around your cigarettes, and you circle the hour you eat, and put an X for the time you wake up and sleep, and a mark for every time you have a cigarette. The first week you have to wait 15 minutes

after every meal before you smoke a cigarette and the second week a half hour, the third week 45 minutes, and the fourth week an hour. I also had to brush my teeth five times a day, and write down every alcoholic or caffeine drink I took.

They never limit your cigarettes, you know, just the times you have them. They make you change brands every week. First you choose a brand you like, other than your regular one, then they make you go to a lower power of nicotine, then to still a lower one. I started with my brand, Marlboro 100s, then I smoked Winston 100s for a week. Then I smoked Tareytons, ones I didn't like. Then I had to smoke Carltons, which is the lowest, I think. I mean, I was glad to give it up when the time came.

They had all kinds of breathing and stretching exercises (I never did them), and you had to look in a mirror and talk to yourself. They gave you a logbook you had to keep. You had to keep a list of the reasons that you wanted to quit smoking, and a list of the things that you want for yourself in life, and every week you had to add to the lists, and read them over every day. They wanted us to drink a quart of water a day, and a couple of glasses of orange juice. They gave us reasons for everything. There were hundreds of things we had to do.

You had a buddy, and a group of four, and every week one person in the group would be captain, and call the other people and see how everyone was doing. You cut out ads for cigarettes and commented on them. They all say how good their brand tastes, but cigarettes don't *taste* good, any of them. The last week we smoked we had to keep a special ashtray, just one, and we saved all the butts from it and put them in a jar. The week after we quit smoking, we all brought our jars into the meeting. Then our leader told us to add a cup of water to the jar and let it sit in our room. I still have mine on my dresser, closed tight.

QUITTING WHILE YOU'RE AHEAD

How fast did you cut down, week by week?
(Pulls out her membership card.) I started at 190 cigarettes, then I went to 125, 108, 106, 15. Some people increased for a while, but at the end almost everybody who stayed in the course had stopped smoking. I remember I went into this bar one day before my cutoff date, and a waiter saw me marking my card, and came over and told me he had quit, and his whole family had quit, and I should really keep on with it.

How do you explain the success of the program? Could you have quit without it?
I'm not sure. The different things we were taught to do—they helped, plus there were all those other people there in the same position I was. I can't explain it. I just know it happened, and that it worked for me.

How about friends of yours who smoked?
Well, my sister quit the same day I did. I suppose she needed someone to tell her a day to quit, and the day I quit, she quit. And the person I'm going out with also quit the same day I did. He had decided he was going to, and I asked him to go to Smokenders with me, but he said he didn't need to.

Have they had trouble?
My sister has. She gained a lot of weight. She really got depressed for a while, too, and I think she's still in a depression. She's 21 now. She smoked 2 packs a day, and she'd been smoking since she was, like, 12 or 13.

Have you recommended the method to your mother?
I know my mother. Even if she was enrolled she would never go.

Has your idea of what you're like changed since you stopped smoking?

I'm very proud I did it. Like when anybody says, "Will you have a cigarette," I'll say, "No, I *quit* smoking." I don't think I'll ever smoke again, because I don't want to.

What was on the list you most wanted for yourself in life?
I want to have, like, five or six children, and, basically, be just a housewife. I want to live in a quiet place, but near the city, probably in Connecticut.

What are you going to do about your children and cigarettes?
I wouldn't want them to smoke, but I know I can't tell them what to do or what not to do. I think that's wrong. Like my mother, I don't see how she has a right—well, she had a *right*, because she's my mother—but telling me not to smoke doesn't mean anything coming from her, because she smokes.

* * *

Most Americans under the age of 25 run such a low risk of death within the decade that standard profiling may give an overly optimistic picture. It tells them, in effect, that their risks are all exterior—that they should worry about motor vehicle accidents and homicide, but not so much about smoking and overeating. The computer, however, can be programmed to project such habits into the 40-year-old range, which is when the invidious effects begin to catch up with people. To do this, the computer adds fifteen or twenty years to the subject's age, then runs his present habits and history through the electronic brain once more. Some processing centers do this automatically for every subject under 35, sending to him or her the long-range prospect at age 40 if present habits are continued, along with the standard ten-year prediction.

In Laura Blake's case, because of her recent habit change, the projection of her statistics forward to the age of 40 does not yield any very dire results. By then she will presumably not have smoked for twenty-one years so her chances against lung and heart disease will be virtually the same as those of someone who never smoked.

Her history is ominously pertinent, however, for the coming generation of middle-aged women. Until recently it is men who have been terrorized by the plague of lung cancer, because it was men as a mass who first took up heavy smoking, starting about sixty years ago. Today the biggest group of new smokers is said to be girls in their teens, who are now smoking at twice the rate of their 1964 counterparts. The expected epidemic of lung cancer has already begun in their mothers and aunts. Last year in Connecticut, for the first time, there were more fatalities from lung cancer among women than among men.

For Laura's health profile, projected forward to age 40, and assuming she remains an ex-smoker, see below.

HEALTH RISK PROFILE

Laura Blake, age 40, white.

Age in terms of present health, 38.

Achievable health age, 37.

An average white woman your age has 2,852 chances per 100,000 of dying in the next ten years; your risks are 16% less than the average. You can, however, reduce these risks by 13%.

FACTORS OFFERING THE GREATEST REDUCTION IN RISK:	THE NUMBER OF YEARS TO BE GAINED BY ALTERING THOSE FACTORS:
Drinking	.6 year
Other factors	.4 year
Total	1.0 years

THE LONGEVITY FACTOR

Your risks of death within the next ten years in descending importance:

1. BREAST CANCER

AVERAGE RISK	342 ●●●●●●●●●●
YOUR CURRENT RISK	274 ●●●●●●●●
YOUR ACHIEVABLE RISK	239 ●●●●●●●

INDICATORS OF RISK	RISK RATING	WAYS TO REDUCE RISK	RISK RATING
Family history of breast cancer—no Monthly self-exam—no Yearly exam by physician—yes	.8	Monthly self-exam—yes	.7

2. CIRRHOSIS OF THE LIVER

AVERAGE RISK	170 ●●●●●●●●●●
YOUR CURRENT RISK	170 ●●●●●●●●●●
YOUR ACHIEVABLE RISK	17 ●

INDICATORS OF RISK	RISK RATING	WAYS TO REDUCE RISK	RISK RATING
Alcohol consumption—7 to 14 drinks per week	1.0	Not drinking	.1
Liver function test not taken—average used	1.0		

3. SUICIDE

AVERAGE RISK	143 ●●●●●●●●●●
YOUR CURRENT RISK	143 ●●●●●●●●●●
YOUR ACHIEVABLE RISK	143 ●●●●●●●●●●

QUITTING WHILE YOU'RE AHEAD

INDICATORS OF RISK	RISK RATING	WAYS TO REDUCE RISK	RISK RATING
Depression—no	1.0		
Family history of suicide—no	1.0		
Alcohol consumption—7 to 14 drinks per week	1.0		

4. CANCER OF THE OVARY

AVERAGE RISK	101 ●●●●●●●●●●
YOUR CURRENT RISK	101 ●●●●●●●●●●
YOUR ACHIEVABLE RISK	101 ●●●●●●●●●●

No risk indicators have been established for this cause of death.

5. LUNG CANCER

AVERAGE RISK	149 ●●●●●●●●●●
YOUR CURRENT RISK	89 ●●●●●●
YOUR ACHIEVABLE RISK	89 ●●●●●●

INDICATORS OF RISK	RISK RATING	WAYS TO REDUCE RISK	RISK RATING
Ex-smoker for more than 5 years	.6		

6. CANCER OF THE LARGE INTESTINE AND RECTUM

AVERAGE RISK	87 ●●●●●●●●●●
YOUR CURRENT RISK	87 ●●●●●●●●●●
YOUR ACHIEVABLE RISK	87 ●●●●●●●●●●

INDICATORS OF RISK	RISK RATING	WAYS TO REDUCE RISK	RISK RATING
Intestinal polyps—none	1.0		

THE LONGEVITY FACTOR

INDICATORS OF RISK	RISK RATING	WAYS TO REDUCE RISK	RISK RATING
Rectal bleeding—none	1.0		
Ulcerative colitis—no	1.0		

7. MOTOR VEHICLE ACCIDENTS

AVERAGE RISK	93 ●●●●●●●●●●
YOUR CURRENT RISK	84 ●●●●●●●●●
YOUR ACHIEVABLE RISK	30 ●●●

INDICATORS OF RISK	RISK RATING	WAYS TO REDUCE RISK	RISK RATING
Alcohol consumption—7 to 14 drinks per week	1.0	No drinks before driving	.5
Mileage—10,000 yearly as driver or passenger	.8		
Seat belt use—less than 10% of time	1.1	Use seat belts always	.8

8. ARTERIOSCLEROTIC HEART DISEASE (heart attack)

AVERAGE RISK	308 ●●●●●●●●●●
YOUR CURRENT RISK	71 ●●
YOUR ACHIEVABLE RISK	57 ●●

INDICATORS OF RISK	RISK RATING	WAYS TO REDUCE RISK	RISK RATING
Current blood pressure 110/60	.4		
Current cholesterol not given—average used	1.0		
Diabetes—none	1.0		
Exercise—some activity	1.0	Exercise—vigorous	.8
Family history of early heart deaths—none	.9		
Former smoker, remain stopped	.8		

QUITTING WHILE YOU'RE AHEAD

INDICATORS OF RISK	RISK RATING	WAYS TO REDUCE RISK	RISK RATING
Weight—115 lbs.	.8		
History of abnormal electrocardiogram— none	1.0		
Current triglycerides not given—average used	1.0		

Excessive stress may increase risk. Exact risk factor not yet available. Use of birth control pills increases risk. Exact risk factor not yet available.

---

9. STROKE

AVERAGE RISK	174 ••••••••••
YOUR CURRENT RISK	70 ••••
YOUR ACHIEVABLE RISK	70 ••••

INDICATORS OF RISK	RISK RATING	WAYS TO REDUCE RISK	RISK RATING
Current blood pressure 110/60	.4		
Current cholesterol not given—average used	1.0		
Diabetes—none	1.0		
Former smoker	1.0		
History of abnormal electrocardiogram— none	1.0		

Use of birth control pills increases risk. Exact risk factor not yet available.

---

10. CANCER OF THE CERVIX

AVERAGE RISK	70 ••••••••••
YOUR CURRENT RISK	55 ••••••••
YOUR ACHIEVABLE RISK	11 ••

THE LONGEVITY FACTOR

INDICATORS OF RISK	RISK RATING	WAYS TO REDUCE RISK	RISK RATING
Economic status—high	.5		
Jewish parentage	.1		
Age of first sexual intercourse—teens	2.5		
Pap smear test—negative within past year	.5	Annual Pap smear in future	.1

OTHER

Your risk of death from all other causes in the next ten years totals 1,215 out of 100,000.

7
QUITTING AFTER IT'S TOO LATE:
Eugene Howell, Smoker

If it's a challenge to give up cigarettes when you're 19, what's it like at the age of 63, after a lifetime of heavy smoking?

"Easy," says Eugene Howell, a trace of irony in his voice. After many previous failures, Gene, a physician by trade, finally quit last year, and attributes his success to desire pure and simple—what behaviorists call "motivation." He says, "This time I didn't *want* to smoke any more. That was all there was to it."

He consumed the last cigarette of his life on the night of January 14, 1977, as a patient in a hospital in Asheville, North Carolina. Dressed in a bathrobe, he slipped out of his room, joined his wife Suzanne in the coffeeshop downstairs, and lit up for one final time. He was to be operated on for lung cancer the following morning.

Why are doctors so drawn to smoking? Probably because of the lives they lead—in a hurry, overworked, under continual stress. This has certainly been true of Gene Howell. Gene studied premed at Yale University (where he first took up smoking at the age of 17), then went on to the College of Physicians and Surgeons at Columbia University, taking his specialty in obstetrics and gynecology. He served in the air force during World War II, then returned to New York and with his young wife, Suzanne, moved into an apartment on the upper East Side, where he was to practice. His prospects were excellent; he could look forward to a successful and highly remunerative career guiding New York's upper-middle-class women through the hazards of childbirth and the menopause.

But he wasn't satisfied.

Howell possesses in abundance certain traits important in the practice of medicine. He is an intelligent and caring man. He is able. He also has considerable personal style—a mixture of wit and authority to which patients respond.

In other ways, however, he differs from many doctors. He is not competitive in the usual sense. There is a questing quality about him, a restlessness concerning aims and goals.

As he set to work, Gene looked around him at the way medicine was being practiced in New York and did not like what he saw: too many doctors, in particular too many specialists (two-thirds of all the medical specialists in the country were practicing in the northeastern states). Gene was well equipped to meet the competition; what bothered him was the point of it all. "Let's say you work hard, and you're lucky, and you rise up the ladder, and one fine day you take over Taylor's position at P and S," he says now (P and S is Columbia's College of Physicians and Surgeons). "That's the pinnacle. Well? So what? The fact is, someone excellent will always get that job. Does it matter whether it's you or some other guy?"

Gene wanted to matter; he wanted to make a difference. In the spring of 1950, aged 34, he took a trip with Suzanne

QUITTING AFTER IT'S TOO LATE

back to Asheville, North Carolina, to visit Suzanne's family. Asheville was a place most unlike New York, a city in the mountains with a population at the time of 53,000. Interested, Howell made inquiries, and also received some: Was he a chiropractor or a licensed physician, someone wanted to know. The question would have been unthinkable in his medical circles up north. But Howell was pleased. A well trained professional could accomplish something in Asheville.

Eight months later he and Suzanne moved south to stay, leaving behind them the glamorous world of big-time urban medicine.

The Howells have spent twenty-eight years in Asheville. There they brought up their two children, formed close and enduring friendships, and lived with a certain style. Gene drove one of the first sports cars in town, a little red Alfa Romeo. A few years later he learned to fly, got a pilot's license, and began renting planes on weekends. But mainly he worked—incredibly hard, as many small-city doctors do. He had his own private practice, with no partner to share calls in the middle of the night. Before long he was working eighty to ninety hours a week and getting his sleep in three-hour snatches. "And it was never the same three hours, that was the worst of it," he remembers. He was also smoking very heavily. How much? Close to three packs a day, he estimates, though he is not really sure: "You see, there weren't any days, just those ninety-hour weeks." Suzanne smoked too; once, on impulse, she quit, and survived quite nicely for three weeks until someone at a cocktail party offered her a cigarette. Gene, when he tried to stop smoking, suffered torments. Even his precious three-hour sleep periods were invaded; he would wake after half an hour, sweating and trembling with the need to smoke. Over a period of years he launched five major crusades to quit, and failed each time. At last he concluded that he was hopelessly addicted, and had better just accept the fact.

He was too busy anyway, or so he thought, to give the matter further attention. At some point he delivered his 6,500th baby, after which he stopped counting. The years passed, one by one. Gene went on smoking.

Captain Eugene Howell, USAF, and Suzanne Brooks met in 1942 in the house of the Episcopal bishop of Nashville, Tennessee. As Gene tells it, "I was 26 years old, a Victorian puritan from up north. And the bishop's daughter-in-law, a schoolmate of a sister of mine, looked at me and said, 'You need a girl.' It embarrassed me. It embarrasses me still." Suzanne, however, was the girl, a beautiful and witty one; ten days later they became engaged, and six months after that they were married.

It has been an unusually strong marriage. Both are favored people—lively, good-looking, socially assured, with a natural capacity for enjoyment. In particular, they enjoy each other. They like and trust each other. While one tells an anecdote, the other listens serenely, smiling in anticipation, though after thirty-seven years of marriage few of the stories can be new. Perhaps they simply enjoy watching each other perform. They are both excellent raconteurs.

Suzanne is tall and blonde, with an easy southern laugh. Gene is of medium height, dark, and intelligent looking. In particular you notice his eyes—alert, warm, with a lurking gleam. He glances at you, you glance at him, and the connection is made. You find yourself beginning to smile.

They have been through good times together. Now they are going through a hard time.

In the autumn of 1976 Gene came down with pneumonia. He got better. Then he came down with bronchitis, which also got better but was followed by a cough that took weeks

QUITTING AFTER IT'S TOO LATE

to clear. Spring came. One Saturday afternoon he went out to hammer some fence posts on his property, developed pain in the chest, and went to see a doctor. The pain, it turned out, was caused by *mediastinitis* and had nothing to do with his lungs. But during the visit a chest X-ray was taken, and a malignant node was discovered.

Only a few years ago lung cancer was treated by surgery when operable; when not, either X-ray therapy or chemotherapy would be attempted. Today, however, a combination of the three techniques is believed to offer the best hope. In Gene's case, the following course of treatment was prescribed:

1. First, two weeks of presurgical radium treatment
2. Surgery, with a week of hospital care
3. Three weeks' recuperation at home
4. Two more weeks of radium
5. Approximately six months of chemotherapy

The program would be long and painful, with little chance of ultimate recovery. At best, only one out of ten patients survives lung cancer for very long.

Gene's prospects sank further when he was operated on. Cancer cells were found in more than one area of his lung, and they were of a particularly malignant type. He describes his prognosis at that point as "very grave, and very brief." Half of his left lung was removed.

Nevertheless, he came home from the hospital and set to work. His doctors had recommended exercise to build his breathing capacity; within a week he was hefting weights, and within three weeks he was riding an exercycle several miles a day. It was very hard for him at first. "You push," he says. "You just keep pushing. It was easy to get off and lie down. And it was hard to get up and go on." Gene kept getting up and going on. He even mowed his lawn one day, somewhat scandalizing his neighbors. He explains, "We live in a neighborhood where the curtains all drop back as you walk down the street. Literally. My first day home from the hospital I went out to pick up the newspaper. It was six-thirty in the morning; I picked up the paper and went back indoors; and the story was all over the neighborhood by ten o'clock."

His hardest times have come with the chemotherapy program. He is getting a set of drugs also used to treat Hodgkin's disease and known as MOPP (a rough acronym for mechlorethamine, vincristine, prednisone, and procarbozine). Every month he is first injected with nitrogen mustard. Then he starts taking pills by mouth (cell killers, he calls them), combined with other medication to counter the side effects—as many as 20 pills a day. The problem is that drugs strong enough to destroy cancer cells will also damage normal tissue, and after two weeks of treatment Gene becomes so debilitated that he must spend a fortnight or longer rebuilding his strength.

During the first month it was his gastrointestinal system that reacted; he suffered nausea, constipation, and pain, and lost 20 pounds.

The second month was worse; he hardly remembers it now, he felt so sick. He lay in bed, unable to eat or drink, his voice reduced to a whisper. "You just sort of faded away," Suzanne says. Gene says, "I was poisoned, was all—plain poisoned. There was no specific thing."

In the third round, however, the effect was highly specific: myocardial toxicity. Gene's heart went into atrial fibrillation and he ended up back in the hospital, in the cardiac care unit. "My heart would beat three or four times, then wait a while, then beat four or five times. That's a lousy feeling." Nevertheless, he pulled himself together and the next day, incredibly, flew off to Syracuse, New York, to attend a medical meeting on a new sterilization

QUITTING AFTER IT'S TOO LATE

program. He is rather proud of this feat, and says it was an excellent and very important meeting.

Howell's treatment for cancer will probably involve a total of six cycles of chemotherapy.

Each time he resumes medication, Gene has to wonder what the side effects are going to be. Most recently his bone marrow was affected, and he developed an anemia so severe that just walking across a room left him gasping for breath. Five weeks later his red-blood-cell count was still only 30 percent of normal, but he was slowly getting around again. One evening he and Suzanne went out to dinner with friends. "The thing that bothers me is this," he said that night. "After five weeks *off* the medication, sure, *I'm* recovering. But what about the cancer, is *it* recovering too? I wouldn't like that a bit."

So he was already bracing himself for his next round of drugs. His mood was determined, yet quite calm. "What else can I do?" he asked. "Oh, I could sit down and just blubber. But where would that get me?"

Sometimes he remembers a movie he saw long ago, about some men on an oil tanker during World War II. In one scene, a sailor is on deck painting a lifeboat, when Nazi planes come in to attack. Eugene describes the vignette: "The sailor is taken by surprise. He hasn't got a chance, and he knows it. So what do you think he does? As the plane comes low, machine guns firing, he takes his paintbrush and he throws it at the airplane. This is the last act of his life. Well, somehow it caught my imagination. And I think now, *That's what I'm doing.*" Gene raises his eyes. Quietly and firmly he says, "I *won't quit*. Even if it doesn't make any sense, I *still* won't quit."

But Gene is convinced that it does make sense, and he is eager for people to understand this. He says that when you suddenly face up to a 10 percent chance of survival, all your attitudes change, and something strange and rather wonderful happens inside you. "What was it Samuel Johnson said, about being sentenced to hang? 'It concentrates the mind.' No, 'It *wonderfully* concentrates the mind.' Johnson was right."

Lung cancer has "concentrated" Gene's mind in ways he still cannot altogether explain. Perhaps they are summed up when he remarks simply, "Good God, it's nice being alive!"

More than halfway through his chemotherapy, Howell has been rewarded with an improved prognosis. Four years of life, his doctors give him now—"four years plus" were the exact words—and Howell is tremendously pleased.

But he has no illusions about his longer-term prospects. He is a physician and a realist, with a trained respect for the capacity of invading malignant cells. He is pleased with his doctors, who he says are not attempting to fit him into some cancer research program but simply trying to save his life, and he follows their directions scrupulously. But he has made up his mind about certain matters.

"I'm going to die at home," he says, "and I'm going to do any plug-pulling that needs to be done, and see that the plug stays pulled." Suzanne, his wife, listens quietly; clearly they have discussed the subject more than once.

Gene has seen a lot of terminal cancer, which he describes as "that utter, horrible, weeks-and-months-long agony and disaster." In his judgment, there is a point past which a kind of minimal decency is lost—"when you're coughing up blood, hemorrhaging, losing weight, you're down to 95 pounds, and all the rest of it. I'm talking about decomposition. Decomposition while you're still alive." At this point, he says, the time has come to go, and death becomes an act that is both rational and constructive for all concerned.

"I feel, what is there? There's love; there's birth; and

there's death," he says, "and we've turned death into something dirty and shameful. This is new, you know. You go visit one of those prerevolutionary graveyards, New England's full of 'em. You'll find whole families: little kids laid out, dead from typhus and diphtheria; wives who died in childbirth; the husbands. And the grandparents. Back in those days you watched the grandparents grow old and fail, it was part of life. Then they died. And you were there. You were what?—five, six, seven years old. The rural life, with all the animals around—that was part of it too. The attitude toward death was healthier, more accepting; death was part of the dialogue. It should have been. It should be today. This is something I want to get across to my own kids."

Howell's son and daughter are in their middle twenties now, both in college working toward degrees after having dropped out during the late 1960s, a troubled time for American youth generally. Howell feels good about the way both of them have responded to his illness. "They don't poop around, they go about their own lives," he says. "But they have expressed just an awful lot of love."

Others have too, and Howell, who says that usually when he's sick "I just want to go under the porch like a dog," feels strangely different now that he is seriously ill. "People seemed to appear from everywhere, out of the woodwork practically," he says. "And it shook me. It does even now. I never will get used to it. Those first days in the hospital, I was—I tell you I had a hard time, I broke down a couple of times. I'm talking about minor, minor forms of support. These suspenders I'm wearing, presented to me by the nurses from my clinic in the mountains, they sent a delegation. And there were others. You just physically feel you're being supported, by something intangible. It's a sense of being held up by hands."

THE LONGEVITY FACTOR

He glances at Suzanne. She smiles at him.

Today Suzanne, too, is an ex-smoker, after thirty-five years on a pack a day. She says, "All those years, it was Gene who kept trying to stop, not me. I was happy smoking. Then he got sick. Of course I had to stop. I had to; there just wasn't any alternative. And I didn't know how.

"He was in the hospital for surgery; I was staying at a motel next door to be near him. It was a very bad time. And all the while, underneath, I kept thinking, *How am I going to stop smoking?*

"He was in intensive care one day, they wouldn't let me visit, so I drove home to pick up some things. Driving back, I suddenly realized I'd left my cigarettes at home. There sat my cigarettes on the mantelpiece, in my living room—and here I was, driving away from them, back to the hospital and Gene.

"It must sound strange, but that was it. That was all there was to it. I just stopped smoking. At that moment, smoking just passed out of my life."

As for that last package of cigarettes, it lay waiting for her the day she brought Gene home, and remained there on the mantel for a period of some months. She liked having it there; somehow its presence reassured her.

Finally she disposed of it. Late one September night, after everyone else was asleep, she took the package out onto the porch and silently chain-smoked for almost an hour in the darkness. She stubbed out the last butt, tossed it into the bushes, and went upstairs to bed.

Today if someone offers Suzanne a cigarette she says "No, thanks," with perfect equanimity. She isn't tempted. Why would she be? She does not want to smoke.

* * *

QUITTING AFTER IT'S TOO LATE

Gene Howell smoked cigarettes for forty-six years, starting at age 17 and quitting at age 63. During most of that time he consumed about 2½ packs a day, and his risk of lung cancer grew steadily, particularly after he entered middle age. Here are the exact figures on which the health profile predictions are based:

Ten-Year Risk of Death from Lung Cancer, per 100,000 Population

	AGE 20	AGE 40	AGE 50	AGE 60
In nonsmokers	.6	70	238	512
In average smokers (½ pack per day)	3.0	348	1,188	2,561
In Howell (more than 2 packs per day)	6.0	696	2,376	5,122

Note that these risks are only for the coming ten years; overall, a heavy smoker has one chance in five of ultimately dying of lung cancer.

Smoking also elevated Gene's risk for heart attack and stroke, particularly since the onset of middle age, when his blood pressure and weight began to rise. In fact, his statistical risk for heart attack was considerably higher than that for lung cancer, as can be seen on the following profile done just before he became ill.

But it was lung cancer that struck Eugene Howell.

HEALTH RISK PROFILE

Eugene Howell, age 63, white.

Age in terms of present health, 75+.

Achievable health age, 68.

An average white man your age has 27,847 chances per 100,000 of dying in the next ten years; your risks are 109% greater than average. You can, however, reduce these risks by 37%.

FACTORS OFFERING THE GREATEST REDUCTION IN RISK:	THE NUMBER OF YEARS TO BE GAINED BY ALTERING THOSE FACTORS:
Weight	2.8 years
Smoking	1.9 years
Blood Pressure	1.7 years
Drinking	.2 year
Other factors	.4 year
Total	7.0 years

Your risks of death within the next ten years in descending importance:

1. ARTERIOSCLEROTIC HEART DISEASE (heart attack)

AVERAGE RISK	11,273 ••••••••••
YOUR CURRENT RISK	32,015 ••••••••••••••••••••••••••••••
YOUR ACHIEVABLE RISK	15,106 •••••••••••••

INDICATORS OF RISK	RISK RATING	WAYS TO REDUCE RISK	RISK RATING
Blood pressure— current, 135/85 average of current and previous:		Blood pressure 120/80 or less	

QUITTING AFTER IT'S TOO LATE

INDICATORS OF RISK	RISK RATING	WAYS TO REDUCE RISK	RISK RATING
Systolic 175	1.8		1.5
Diastolic 97	1.4		1.3
Current cholesterol not given—average used	1.0		
Diabetes—none	1.0		
Exercise—vigorous	.6		
Family history of early heart deaths—none	.9		
Smoker—2 packs per day	1.3	Not smoking	1.0
Weight 263 lbs.	1.8	Reduce to 169 lbs. or less	1.0
History of abnormal electrocardiogram—none	1.0		
Triglycerides not given—average used	1.0		

Excessive stress may increase risk. Exact risk factor not yet available.

2. LUNG CANCER

AVERAGE RISK	2,561 ●●●●●●●●●●
YOUR CURRENT RISK	7,683 ●●●●●●●●●●●●●●●●●●●●●●●●●●●●
YOUR ACHIEVABLE RISK	6,146 ●●●●●●●●●●●●●●●●●●●●●●●●

INDICATORS OF RISK	RISK RATING	WAYS TO REDUCE RISK	RISK RATING
Smoker—2 packs per day	3.0	Not smoking	2.4
		Remain stopped 8 years	?

3. STROKE

AVERAGE RISK	1,775 ●●●●●●●●●●
YOUR CURRENT RISK	4,260 ●●●●●●●●●●●●●●●●●●●●●●●●
YOUR ACHIEVABLE RISK	3,195 ●●●●●●●●●●●●●●●●●●

THE LONGEVITY FACTOR

INDICATORS OF RISK	RISK RATING	WAYS TO REDUCE RISK	RISK RATING
Blood pressure—average of current and previous:		Blood pressure 120/80 or less	
Systolic 175	1.8		1.5
Diastolic 97	1.4		1.3
Current cholesterol not given—average used	1.0		
Diabetes—none	1.0		
Smoker—2 packs per day	1.2	Not smoking	1.0
History of abnormal electrocardiogram—none	1.0		

4. BRONCHITIS AND EMPHYSEMA

AVERAGE RISK	736 ••••••••••
YOUR CURRENT RISK	2,208 ••••••••••••••••••••••••••••••
YOUR ACHIEVABLE RISK	1,546 ••••••••••••••••••••••

INDICATORS OF RISK	RISK RATING	WAYS TO REDUCE RISK	RISK RATING
Smoker—2 packs per day	3.0	Not smoking	2.1
Lung function test normal	1.0		

5. CIRRHOSIS OF THE LIVER

AVERAGE RISK	693 ••••••••••
YOUR CURRENT RISK	832 ••••••••••••
YOUR ACHIEVABLE RISK	69 •

INDICATORS OF RISK	RISK RATING	WAYS TO REDUCE RISK	RISK RATING
Alcohol consumption—15 to 24 drinks per week	1.2	Not drinking	.1
Liver function test normal	1.0		

6. CANCER OF THE LARGE INTESTINE AND RECTUM

AVERAGE RISK	814 ●●●●●●●●●●
YOUR CURRENT RISK	814 ●●●●●●●●●●
YOUR ACHIEVABLE RISK	244 ●●●

INDICATORS OF RISK	RISK RATING	WAYS TO REDUCE RISK	RISK RATING
Intestinal polyps—none	1.0		
Rectal bleeding—none	1.0		
Ulcerative colitis—none	1.0		
Annual sigmoidoscopy— none	1.0	Annual in future	.3

7. DISEASES OF THE ARTERIES

AVERAGE RISK	284 ●●●●●●●●●●
YOUR CURRENT RISK	682 ●●●●●●●●●●●●●●●●●●●●●●●●
YOUR ACHIEVABLE RISK	511 ●●●●●●●●●●●●●●●●●●

INDICATORS OF RISK	RISK RATING	WAYS TO REDUCE RISK	RISK RATING
Blood pressure—average of current and previous:		Blood pressure 120/80 or less	
Systolic 175	1.8		1.5
Diastolic 97	1.4		1.3
Current cholesterol not given—average used	1.0		
Diabetes—none	1.0		
Smoker 2 packs per day	1.2	Not smoking	1.0

8. PNEUMONIA

AVERAGE RISK	483 ●●●●●●●●●●
YOUR CURRENT RISK	580 ●●●●●●●●●●●●
YOUR ACHIEVABLE RISK	483 ●●●●●●●●●●

THE LONGEVITY FACTOR

INDICATORS OF RISK	RISK RATING	WAYS TO REDUCE RISK	RISK RATING
Alcohol consumption—15 to 24 drinks per week	1.0		
No history of bacterial pneumonia	1.0		
No history of emphysema	1.0		
Smoker—2 packs per day	1.2	Not smoking	1.0
Lung function test normal	1.0		

9. CANCER OF THE PROSTATE

AVERAGE RISK	422 ••••••••••
YOUR CURRENT RISK	422 ••••••••••
YOUR ACHIEVABLE RISK	295 •••••••

INDICATORS OF RISK	RISK RATING	WAYS TO REDUCE RISK	RISK RATING
Annual rectal exam—none	1.0	Annual in future	.7

10. SUICIDE

AVERAGE RISK	289 ••••••••••
YOUR CURRENT RISK	289 ••••••••••
YOUR ACHIEVABLE RISK	289 ••••••••••

INDICATORS OF RISK	RISK RATING	WAYS TO REDUCE RISK	RISK RATING
Depression—none	1.0		
Family history of suicide—none	1.0		
Alcohol consumption—15 to 24 drinks per week	1.0		

OTHER

Your risk of death from all other causes in the next ten years totals 8,517 out of 100,000.

8

TRYING:
Lucille Meeker, Overeater

"About the time breakfast is over I usually think, *Now what am I going to have for lunch?*" says Lucille Meeker, smiling a big, rueful smile. She is a 41-year-old black woman with bright eyes and a warm voice. Lucille sees the humor in life—even in the personal problem that has been plaguing her for 25 years now, and which she is seemingly incapable of solving. In this she is not alone: between 40 and 80 million Americans are obese, and it is estimated that 95 percent of them will remain so for the rest of their lives, except for brief periods when they embark on crash diets.

Lucille first became overweight in her teens. Today she isn't sure what she weighs—she says her scale wasn't accurate, so she got rid of it—but probably well up in the 160s. She is only 5' 1½" tall.

Oddly, you don't notice her condition at first glance. Her face, chin, and neck are slim and firm; her upper torso is normal. She is one of those people whose extra poundage all settles in the hips and thighs, and these she has learned to camouflage. Greeting visitors in her apartment not long ago, she wore a long sleeveless coat, made of cotton and tan in color, over a dark flowered shirt and plain pants. She looked attractive, certainly anything but obese.

Lucille has been using coats for years to conceal her problem. In college at Tuskegee Institute, she says, she always kept a coat on in social places such as the cafeteria or student union, no matter what the temperature, and used to get kidded for it. Once, as a joke, a boy she knew came up from behind, suddenly pulled the coat off her, and began tossing it back and forth with a group of friends. Lucille felt like going through the floor with embarrassment.

Today the only person likely to tease her is her husband Wayne. He does needle her frequently.

Wayne is a cheerful, trimly built man with a West Indies accent—he grew up on the island of Barbados. He and Lucille met at Tuskegee, where he studied accounting. Today he works as manager of a small supermarket. Lucille is a teacher in a Head Start program for three- to five-year-olds. The Meekers have three children of their own, and live in a suburb of Cleveland, Ohio, just across the city line—a well kept community with a good public school system. One senses they are people on the way up in the world—friendly, confident, ambitious, with strong hopes for their children.

Life for Lucille Meeker would be good indeed, if she could just conquer her weight problem. It isn't only her appearance she's concerned about. Her mother, who was also obese, died of a blood clot at the age of 52, and two of her brothers were killed by heart attacks, one at 48, the other at 49. Lucille has had kidney problems and today functions on only one kidney, the other having been surgically removed fourteen years ago. Obesity is hard on both the heart and the kidneys.

Lucille by now has tried just about all the weight-loss programs ever invented and can tell you in detail about each one. She has been on the Stillman diet, on the Atkins diet, on pills, and on liquid protein. She has also been a member of several groups.

But only once has she succeeded in losing weight steadily over a protracted period: in 1975, when she joined Weight Watchers, where she lasted six months and shed a total of 25 pounds. This brought her down to 142, more than halfway to her goal weight of 125—strong encouragement, surely, to remain in the program.

Then why did she drop out? Lucille does her best to answer the question. There were problems with Weight Watchers, she says. It was wintertime. The roads were icy. So she decided to drop the meetings for a while and follow the diet by herself, now that she knew how. All went well for a few weeks. Then difficulties began. Weight Watchers had taught her to weigh the food she ate, to make sure she wasn't taking too much of anything; away from the group, she stopped this practice, confident that her eye was as good a judge of quantity as the scale had been. Perhaps it really wasn't, she now concedes.

She also began violating another Weight Watchers tenet: eating slowly.

"I'd give the family their dinner," she remembers. "Then I'd fix something for myself, and sit down with it. I was supposed to eat a forkful of food, put the fork down, maybe read or talk, then eat another forkful. Well, everything got off schedule: getting my little girl to bed; checking the boys' homework. I haven't got that kind of time.

"And I don't like eating alone. And if you eat alone, you might eat more. But if you eat with the family, you might eat fast."

It was during this period, too, that she threw away her faulty scales; after that, she could no longer keep track of her weight.

What else? Lucille pauses, searching her memory. A smile appears at the corners of her mouth. She confesses,

"One day I had me a dish of ice cream. Maple walnut. I asked myself, 'Why not?' I had lost 25 pounds. Everyone was saying to me, 'You're so skinny!' and, 'Oooh, my! don't you look fabulous!' Just one dish, I said to myself. It was a mistake."

Lucille doesn't just want to lose pounds. She would also like to cut back on cholesterol, sugar, and other substances she believes to be deleterious to the health of the whole family. She would especially like to deemphasize meat in the menu.

"Steak!" she says. "My husband'll sit there, slicing it. The kids'll say, 'Daddy, may I have another serving?' Later I'll say to him, 'Wayne, next time let's make the steak a little smaller.' He doesn't agree. He says, 'No, meat is important.'

"Well, I've been trying to stress to him that meat is *not* that important, that you can substitute, have macaroni and cheese one day and not have that meat. But my kids don't like macaroni and cheese. They like pizza—something that to me is not nutritious."

Lucille reports that one night she fixed macaroni and cheese for dinner. "I put it on the table. They said, 'Mommy, where's the meat?'

"I said, 'This is the meat tonight. It's protein, a good substitute.'

" 'But we don't like it!'

" 'Well, there isn't anything else. Either you eat this, or you don't eat anything.' And so they didn't eat anything!" cries Lucille, bursting into laughter. "Of course my husband was furious. He said, 'I told you! I told you always to serve meat!' "

Food is tied closely to Lucille's memories of the past—for instance, trying to establish the time of her kidney operation, she'll say, "It must have been November, because I couldn't fix the turkey that year."

She also remembers the food of her childhood. Lucille grew up in Clarksdale, Mississippi, one of seven children of a minister in the Church of Christ. In those days people believed that hearty eating was a sign of good health. "I remember my mother piling our plates up, saying, 'Now eat all that food!' We were a big family. We'd sit around the table, and there'd be a platter of chicken in the middle. We'd be sitting there, enjoying the chicken. But there'd be maybe one or two pieces left on the platter—and all the kids were trying to finish to get those extra pieces of chicken. You always tried to eat fast so as to get seconds."

The youngest in the family, Lucille remembers herself as pert and outspoken, the only one who would stand up to her rigorously strict father when he laid down the law. Surprisingly often she got her way—perhaps her father responded to her fearlessness with a special affection. Nevertheless, she received her share of whippings, and there were periods in her childhood when it seemed she was always in trouble. When she got upset, she'd eat something.

Lucille still eats when upset, but what upsets her the most these days is her eating problem; thus she is caught in a vicious cycle.

She keeps trying.

Last summer she was invited to a family reunion back in Clarksdale; she decided she just *had* to get her weight down, at least part way. And she did. She discovered that a friend of hers had just gone into the dieting business, selling a weight-loss package consisting of a month's supply of liquid protein, plus vitamin, iron, and potassium pills, and including a book, *The Last Chance Diet*. Lucille bought.

In the ensuing weeks Lucille consumed nothing but the

liquid protein, the pills, and an occasional can of diet soda. The pounds began to fall away. She was feeling pretty good about herself. And yet . . . and yet. . . . Back from Clarksdale, she began worrying. Could it be healthy, never eating anything solid, consuming nothing but manmade chemicals? Within a week Lucille was back on 100 percent real food.

She next decided that exercise might help her. It was summertime. Every night after dinner she and her children would go out. "They were really helping me," she recalls. "I'd walk. They would jog. Every night I'd walk around the block, walk religiously, working up to the point where I'd be able to jog too."

But that's when the problems arose. She explains, "You see, I stopped going out because to run, I needed sneakers. So I stopped for a night or two. Told the kids, 'When I get me my sneakers, I'll be back out.' And, you know, they had their friends come knock on the door: 'Mrs. Meeker, you ready to go? We're going round the block.' It was nice, it was really nice. My own kids: 'Mommy, come on, wear your regular shoes and you can walk.' But I wanted to run. I felt I had walked, and built up my strength, and that I was ready. So I stayed home one night, and then I stayed home again the next night. . . ."

A week later Lucille had a fall, breaking a bone in her left foot. The foot was put in a cast, and at this point Lucille, now on crutches, went off to a shoestore and bought sneakers, which today sit on the floor of her closet, waiting for her foot to finish healing. The other night one of her sons asked, "Mommy, you going to start jogging when your foot's better?"

"I said, 'Oh, you bet!' " reports Lucille. "And my husband said, '*Plus*, lose some weight!' "

Lucille wishes someone would *make* her lose—maybe her doctor. "If he'd only come out and say, 'Lucille, you're going to die if you go on eating like this, but if you cut down you're going to live a long time: you decide'—well, I think I'd be able to do it," she says, a little wistfully. "I do believe my eating is going to shorten my life—I do. But I have to be told that.

"For instance, this foot doctor. I saw him yesterday. And I was waiting for him to say to me, 'You're overweight, and that's why your foot is healing so slowly'— because it *is* healing slowly—but he didn't say anything. So *I* mentioned it. He said, 'Oh, you're healthy.' I got mad at him! I said, 'How can you sit there and tell me I'm healthy! I'm too fat!' He said, 'If you're too fat, then lose some weight!'

"Why didn't he say at the very beginning, 'Now Mrs. Meeker, you've got to lose 40 pounds. Starting today, I want you to work on it'?"

But the only person who presses Lucille to lose is Wayne, her husband, and the effect is not helpful. It's the way he says it, Lucille believes. "You know, he'll say, 'Why are you eating that! You *know* what it's going to do to you!'" Lucille finds herself retaliating, as she admits, sneaking into the kitchen when she thinks he won't notice. "I'm only hurting myself. I know that," she says. "But I'm angry."

Lucille won't even tell Wayne what she weighs—or rather, what she weighed at the time she threw away her scales last year. She'll tell a visitor, though, once Wayne has left the apartment. The door closes behind him, and Lucille, her eyes conspiratorial, leans forward and whispers, "One hundred and sixty-seven!" She bursts out laughing. Then she wipes her eyes, sighs, murmurs, "Oh my goodness."

Sometimes when Lucille is restless or upset, she changes her apartment around; in her attempt to stay away from the refrigerator, she'll start moving furniture. "My husband'll come in, he'll say, 'You moved the furniture again! *Why did you move the furniture!*' Then there'll be an argument. So what can I do? I go into the kitchen. While I'm in there he'll come in, still talking about the furniture. All the time, I'm thinking about food. I'm looking in the refrigerator. And I'm finding things, oh . . ."

Lucille's most recent attempt involved yet another liquid protein, one she bought over the counter in a drugstore. It is called *Nature Slim*. "It's a powder," says Lucille. "You mix it with your skimmed milk, or with whatever you're drinking, and that's your meal. But at dinnertime you can have a regular dinner.

"I took it yesterday. And I was doing beautifully till about one o'clock. At one o'clock I went into the kitchen. I figured I'd put this stuff in some milk, make it into a milkshake.

"All of a sudden I thought, *I don't want it! Why should I swallow this stuff! I'm going to have me a nice meal!*

"I found myself eating, and eating, and eating. I really wasn't that hungry, but I just couldn't stop. You see, it's psychological.

"First I was going to make a salad. Then I realized I didn't have the kind of salad dressing that I prefer, I didn't have the vinegar—you see, I mix vinegar with just a little mayonnaise and some ketchup. So I decided not to have that. Instead, I had soup, chicken noodle soup, and I decided I would only have a small cup instead of a bowl. But when I was finished I said, 'Gee, that soup was so good! Maybe I'll have another cup.' Then I wanted toast with it. So I had the toast with the soup.

"Did I butter that toast? I sure did. It just didn't seem right not to. I ate three slices of toast—I don't know, I was just like a vacuum.

"All the time I knew there was some cake up on one of the kitchen shelves. And after I'd eaten the three slices of toast I asked myself, *What else can I eat?*—Just like I was looking for it!

"Then I realized what I was doing, and I came out of the kitchen. I knew if I could get out of the kitchen, maybe I could stop thinking about food. But then the phone rang.

"Now I have a phone in the bedroom. But the phone that I ran to was the one in the kitchen. In the process of talking on the phone—I cut a slice of cake! I sat there, eating cake and talking to my girlfriend. It wasn't till after that last piece, and I was finished, and I was drinking some pineapple juice, that I began feeling very bad. By then it was too late.

"That was yesterday. Today I had some peach yogurt for lunch. That was all. Hopefully I won't . . . I'm really not hungry today. I haven't had time to think about food today."

Though discouraged, Lucille has never become seriously depressed over her problem; she believes this is because she is an open kind of person who does not suppress her feelings. "Something's bothering me, I'll say so," she says. "If someone comes to the house and Wayne and I have quarreled, I just lay it on the line, I tell 'em, 'We're mad, but don't worry, we'll come round eventually.' And, sure enough, we will.

"Now if the children aren't doing as well as they should in school, my husband'll get up tight. But I try to keep a calm attitude. I'll say, 'You know, no one is perfect.'

"And maybe I'll bring out a pencil with a big eraser. I'll tell the kids, 'You know why they put this eraser on this pencil? Because they know we all make a mistake sometimes. But that doesn't mean it has to *remain* a mistake. You can erase it—and start all over again. It's not too late!' I say, 'You know, you always learn from your failures—learn not to do that again.' "

* * *

When Lucille's health profile came in the mail her first reaction was relief. Despite the fact that she is seriously overweight, her overall health risk for the coming ten years was almost exactly average. She must be doing something right.

Then she studied the profile more closely. She discovered that out of the ten listed causes of death, her risk for six was actually lower than average. This is mainly because she neither smokes nor drinks.

But with the good news came some bad: just as she suspected, Lucille's risk for cardiovascular disease was high: 1.8 times the average for heart attack, and 1.5 times the average for hypertensive heart disease.

The reasons are almost all calorie-related: too much food, too little exercise. Lucille not only weighs too much. Her blood pressure and cholesterol are also on the high side, as they so often are in obese, sedentary people.

Proper diet and exercise could reduce Lucille's odds for a heart attack by two-thirds—down to a negligible 626 out of 100,000, and lower her risk age to 38.

Here is her health profile in detail:

HEALTH RISK PROFILE

Lucille Meeker, age 41, black.

Age in terms of present health, 41.

Achievable health age, 38.

An average black woman your age has 6,344 chances per 100,000 of dying in the next ten years; your risks are 1% less than the average. You can, however, reduce these risks by 24%.

TRYING

FACTORS OFFERING THE GREATEST REDUCTION IN RISK:	THE NUMBER OF YEARS TO BE GAINED BY ALTERING THOSE FACTORS:
Weight	1.0 year
Exercise	.8 year
Blood pressure	.7 year
Cholesterol	.3 year
Other factors	.2 year
Total	3.0 years

Your risks of death within the next ten years in descending importance:

1. ARTERIOSCLEROTIC HEART DISEASE (heart attack)

AVERAGE RISK	1,061 ●●●●●●●●●●
YOUR CURRENT RISK	1,931 ●●●●●●●●●●●●●●●●●●●
YOUR ACHIEVABLE RISK	626 ●●●●●●

INDICATORS OF RISK	RISK RATING	WAYS TO REDUCE RISK	RISK RATING
Current blood pressure 140/90	1.0	Blood pressure 120/80 or lower	.7
Current cholesterol 220	.9	Cholesterol 180 or lower	.7
Diabetes—none	1.0		
Exercise—sedentary	1.4	Exercise—moderate	1.0
Family history of early heart deaths—one parent	1.2		
Nonsmoker	.8		
Weight 169 lbs	1.5	Weight 114 lbs. or less	1.0
History of abnormal electrocardiogram—none	1.0		
Current triglycerides 150	1.0		

Excessive stress may increase risk. Exact risk factor not yet available.

THE LONGEVITY FACTOR

2. STROKE

AVERAGE RISK	597 ●●●●●●●●●●
YOUR CURRENT RISK	376 ●●●●●●●
YOUR ACHIEVABLE RISK	263 ●●●●

INDICATORS OF RISK	RISK RATING	WAYS TO REDUCE RISK	RISK RATING
Current blood pressure 140/90	1.0	Blood pressure 120/80 or less	.7
Current cholesterol 220	.9		
Diabetes—none	1.0		
Nonsmoker	.7		
History of abnormal electrocardiogram—none	1.0		

3. BREAST CANCER

AVERAGE RISK	404 ●●●●●●●●●●
YOUR CURRENT RISK	283 ●●●●●●●●
YOUR ACHIEVABLE RISK	283 ●●●●●●●●

INDICATORS OF RISK	RISK RATING	WAYS TO REDUCE RISK	RISK RATING
Family history of breast cancer—none			
Monthly self-examination—yes	.7		
Yearly exam by physician—yes			

TRYING

4. HOMICIDE

AVERAGE RISK	196 ●●●●●●●●●●
YOUR CURRENT RISK	196 ●●●●●●●●●●
YOUR ACHIEVABLE RISK	196 ●●●●●●●●●●

INDICATORS OF RISK	RISK RATING	WAYS TO REDUCE RISK	RISK RATING
No arrests for violence	1.0		
Does not carry weapon	1.0		
Nondrinker	1.0		

5. HYPERTENSIVE HEART DISEASE

AVERAGE RISK	128 ●●●●●●●●●●
YOUR CURRENT RISK	192 ●●●●●●●●●●●●●●●
YOUR ACHIEVABLE RISK	90 ●●●●●●●

INDICATORS OF RISK	RISK RATING	WAYS TO REDUCE RISK	RISK RATING
Current blood pressure 140/90	1.0	Blood pressure 120/80 or less	.7
Weight 169 lbs.	1.5	Weight 114 lbs. or less	1.0

6. PNEUMONIA

AVERAGE RISK	143 ●●●●●●●●●●
YOUR CURRENT RISK	143 ●●●●●●●●●●
YOUR ACHIEVABLE RISK	143 ●●●●●●●●●●

INDICATORS OF RISK	RISK RATING	WAYS TO REDUCE RISK	RISK RATING
Nondrinker	1.0		
No history of bacterial pneumonia	1.0		
No history of emphysema	1.0		
Nonsmoker	1.0		

THE LONGEVITY FACTOR

7. LUNG CANCER

AVERAGE RISK	194 ●●●●●●●●●●
YOUR CURRENT RISK	116 ●●●●●●
YOUR ACHIEVABLE RISK	116 ●●●●●●

INDICATORS OF RISK	RISK RATING	WAYS TO REDUCE RISK	RISK RATING
Nonsmoker	.6		

8. NEPHRITIS AND NEPHROSIS

AVERAGE RISK	104 ●●●●●●●●●●
YOUR CURRENT RISK	104 ●●●●●●●●●●
YOUR ACHIEVABLE RISK	104 ●●●●●●●●●●

No risk indicators have been established for this cause of death.

9. CIRRHOSIS OF THE LIVER

AVERAGE RISK	468 ●●●●●●●●●●
YOUR CURRENT RISK	47 ●
YOUR ACHIEVABLE RISK	47 ●

INDICATORS OF RISK	RISK RATING	WAYS TO REDUCE RISK	RISK RATING
Nondrinker	.1		
Liver function test not taken—average assumed	1.0		

TRYING

10. CANCER OF THE CERVIX

AVERAGE RISK	182 ●●●●●●●●●●
YOUR CURRENT RISK	47 ●●●
YOUR ACHIEVABLE RISK	24 ●

INDICATORS OF RISK	RISK RATING	WAYS TO REDUCE RISK	RISK RATING
Economic status—medium	.6		
History of intercourse	1.7		
Pap smear—3 negative Pap smears in past 5 years	.2	Annual Pap smear in future	.1

OTHER

Your risk of death from all other causes in the next ten years totals 2,867 out of 100,000.

9
A STRENUOUS MENU:
Ed Solomon, Angina Patient

Edwin Solomon is very fond of his mother, with but one reservation: "Feeding is the way she shows love, and for her the best kind of love is always high-fat—you know, the Jewish Mother," he says, smiling a little. "Well, I was the Jewish son. Butter, meat, cheese cake, sour cream. Those were the foods I grew up on. Unfortunately, they became my pattern."

Solomon's Jewish father died a decade ago of heart failure, after suffering acutely from angina, a very painful condition in which the coronary arteries become clogged, depriving the heart of oxygen. Four years ago Ed himself, at the age of 43, began to show signs of the same crippling malady. He did not tell his mother about it. He did not tell anyone except his wife. He felt ashamed and afraid of the disabling pain: "I thought people would say, 'Look at that poor guy over there with angina.' "

Today Ed still has angina, but he has been able to bring it under control through a program of rigid diet and simple exercise, and there is a possibility of curing the condition

A STRENUOUS MENU

entirely. Most doctors say this can be done only by surgery, but personal experience has made Ed more hopeful.

One recent evening he discussed his illness in the living room of his home in suburban Chicago, a comfortable room that shows only some of the scruff of bringing up the Solomons' three energetic sons. Thin, almost frail looking as a result of a recent loss in weight, he sat slightly huddled in his leather lounge chair, the classic tired businessman at the end of a long day, drained but unemotional, surviving. By profession he is an engineer with a secure job in factory construction, a job he is tired of.

Several years ago, rounding the age of 40, Solomon was confidently fleshy—185 pounds compared with his current 147. During that earlier period of his life he was too busy, or so he believed, to get much exercise—only a little swimming in the summer, and an hour or two of tennis on weeks when he could fit it in.

The subject of tennis holds a certain irony for him. At the time he began ailing with angina, he had just finished construction of a commercial four-court tennis club, an intricate business undertaking that had kept him harried over the course of many months. He had built the club as a business sideline, but also because he himself likes to play tennis. And it was at the completed club, playing, that he suffered his first angina attack. "It's a strange feeling," he says, "hard to describe if you haven't experienced it: nauseous, a squeezing feeling, out of breath, a feeling as if you've overeaten. I stopped playing for a few minutes and it went away. Then I played again, and it came back."

A few days later, on his way to work, ascending the stairs from the parking lot to his office, he found himself completely out of breath. "Just one flight of stairs. . . . I decided I'd better see a doctor."

His family physician, an internist, drew a blank. After

117

giving Ed an electrocardiogram to trace his heart action and finding no irregularity, he told him he was simply a little out of condition; perhaps he should go out and do some jogging. But Ed had a heart specialist friend who, hearing his symptoms, said the cause could be angina. The cardiologist sent him to a local hospital for a stress test—an ECG administered while the patient runs on a treadmill. Solomon got up to only 105 pulse beats per minute before his symptoms began and the machine reacted. It was angina, all right.

The first treatment for this malady is usually drugs which dilate the arteries, allowing more blood to flow through to the heart. Solomon started out on Inderal four times a day plus nitroglycerine during attacks of pain. But over the next two years larger and larger doses became necessary as his coronary arteries continued to clog. In 1977 his cardiologist recommended an exploratory operation called an angiogram, in which a small tube is inserted into one of the coronary arteries. Dye is injected, and X-ray motion pictures are taken of the blood as it flows toward the heart. Solomon's report was alarming; two of his three coronary arteries were 85 to 90 percent blocked, the third one 50 percent blocked. His heart was not getting enough blood to support even the exertion of a brisk walk. The angiogram specialist told Solomon he was living dangerously, and strongly recommended a double-bypass operation.

The coronary bypass has, in the past decade, become a standard form of surgery, although it remains complicated, relatively perilous, and very expensive (usually above $10,000). In this procedure a section of healthy vein is taken from another part of the patient's body, and its two ends are spliced into the blocked artery on either side of the blockage. The blood then flows around the block. Not all cardiologists have complete confidence that this leads to greater longevity, however; some studies indicate that the

A STRENUOUS MENU

new bypass arteries often develop blockages of their own. Solomon's friendly cardiologist was one of the doubters. Solomon felt reluctant too. "There was something about the bypass that didn't sound right to me," he says. "In engineering, we'd call it a dirty fix: you know, when something basic is wrong with your design, but instead of fixing it then and there on the drawing board, you bypass, you get around it some way. You can make the thing go for a while that way, but eventually the original problem comes back and stops you."

Yet Solomon had to do something. As he became increasingly incapacitated, he was also becoming seriously depressed. "It seemed as if things were being taken away from me one by one: swimming, tennis, sex." Just walking down the street now, he needed to stop and rest every few steps.

And increasingly, as the months passed, Solomon found himself *not* stopping, pushing on despite his pain and breathlessness, taking chances. "You can do that with angina," he says, "work your way through the pain and out the other side, in effect. Apparently the arteries stretch a little, if your heart keeps pumping. It's like blowing up a balloon, hard at first, then easier after you get some air in it."

If your heart keeps pumping.

Decisions for or against optional surgery are always difficult, especially for someone of Ed's temperament. As an engineer, he's used to making decisions based on facts, preferably "*all* the facts, lined up in front of you. You look them over, and see that they fit together in a systematic way, and your choice becomes obvious. But if some of the facts are missing, then you've got to make a judgment on your own. That's when I start waking up at four in the morning and worrying.

"I'd lie there. I'd think, *Maybe if I hold off for a year or two, they'll develop something safer than a bypass—a Roto-Rooter for arteries, maybe.* In which case I should just increase my drug prescription again and wait. Another night, maybe I'd have had a bad time with my wife. I'd say to myself, *The hell with it, I'll go have the operation.*"

But before a final decision became necessary, Solomon discovered an alternative. He read a magazine article about a man named Nathan Pritikin who was running a clinic in California for sufferers from angina and other cardiovascular problems. The article was so enthusiastic Solomon asked a California friend to investigate the clinic for him. The friend's report was favorable. So, on the whole, was the reaction of his cardiologist. "Try it," he said. "What have you got to lose?" The month with Pritikin would be expensive, $3,500 plus air fare, eating up most of Ed's uncommitted capital. But he was persuaded. He packed his angina pills, and in the bitter cold January of 1977 took a plane to Santa Barbara. Here is what happened there, in his words:

> The first thing that hit me was the weather, just gorgeous, especially coming from Chicago that particular January. . . .
>
> Pritikin and his people had taken over this hotel in Santa Barbara and converted it to medical labs, plus rooms for the patients to stay in. It overlooked the ocean. My group was about 86 patients and 20 husbands and wives, the most people they had ever had for the one-month program. The clinic at that time had been running less than a year.
>
> That first night we ate a regular meal, the kind of food most Americans have for dinner. But the next day we went on the Pritikin regimen, which breaks your eating down into eight separate "meals" a day, with exercise immediately following

A STRENUOUS MENU

each of them. There were blood tests and other tests to be taken along the way.

Pritikin's whole idea is to lower the fats in the blood, both the cholesterol and the triglycerides. His diet is so severe it is more a *no* fat diet than a *low* fat diet, well beyond the American Heart Association recommendations. The AHA diet allows you about 35 percent of your calories in fat, and Pritikin's is no more than 10 percent. He is against all the fats, including the polyunsaturateds. It is not a Jewish mother's menu.

We ate light meals of complex carbohydrates—vegetables, and fruit, bran. No butter, no cheese, no meat, no refined sugar, no milk, no eggs. No salt either, no tea or coffee. No alcohol, of course, Then we would go walking.

Most doctors recommend you walk *before* meals, but Pritikin has his own theories. His idea is to spread out the digestive process through the whole day; you walk after meals to divert blood from your stomach into your legs, and digest slowly, so as not to hit your system with any kind of overload.

I started off by walking down the block and back—slowly. That was all I was capable of. But it surprised me how fast the situation changed. At the beginning I was still taking drugs—you have to go off them very gradually. The clinic doctors were extremely careful, dropping the dosage a little bit each week, or half week. On the walking I progressed rapidly, until after two weeks I was capable of going as far as I wanted to. I also increased my pace as the program went along. Sometimes we would take what they called a meal with us, which might be an orange, and eat it while we were out there, and continue walking.

The rest of the time we would just relax, and it was a really nice relaxation. It was away from work, and all the stress levels were down. As I've said, I'm involved with these tennis courts, a second job for me and often quite a headache.

Every night Pritikin delivered a lecture, during which he was under constant questioning. He was able, in my opinion, to handle anything that was thrown at him and come back without sounding as if he was glossing anything over. He's quiet, soft spoken, with time for everybody, although he is very busy. Pritikin was originally an inventor; he has about twenty patents to his name. He had angina himself when he was in his forties, and the doctors didn't offer any hope. So he went on a research mission. He compiled a record of all the tests and studies that had been made, and came up with this program. He says he cured himself of angina. I know he's in his mid-sixties, and he runs around like a 25-year-old boy. He's not a doctor himself, though he has several doctors on his staff.

We had people out there who'd had heart attacks, bypass surgery, all kinds of circulatory problems—also a woman in her forties with a bad case of stomach ulcers. They all seemed to improve. One fellow had a minor heart attack while we were there; that was the only medical problem that developed that I know about.

There were some who were not sick, a number of them younger people. One girl was just married, and her husband had to be away, so she checked into the program to learn the right way to live. We had a man there who was 92, nothing wrong with him, a sprightly little fellow. He just wanted to attend. He was a multimillionaire. He made something like $800,000 just in interest the previous year. He'd show me his brokerage reports and ask what should he do. You know: problems.

Even before Santa Barbara, Ed had gone on a low-fat diet, reducing his cholesterol reading from 300 to 225; in the month with Pritikin, he succeeded in dropping it to 160. His weight went from 170 to 158. He was walking a dozen miles a day, and had entirely given up medication. He went home full of trepidation that this progress would pass. But by continuing the regimen—taking fatless soups and an orange to the office in the morning, walking before work in

A STRENUOUS MENU

his neighborhood, walking again on a golf course near the office at lunchtime, and again near home in the evening—he has continued to make progress.

His first weeks back home his only problem was periods of dizziness, with dropping blood pressure. Finally one day he telephoned the clinic long distance. "Of course I had already finished the course, and Pritikin was busy with others. But he called me back and spent twenty minutes asking questions, talking to me about the whole thing. At last he told me to take more food, and that seemed to do the trick."

What Ed has not yet succeeded in doing, quite, is in lowering his cholesterol count to the magic Pritikin value, 150, at which point, Pritikin believes, the buildup of fats in the arteries actually commences to reverse itself. The theory is that the body needs cholesterol, and if it's not available in the diet it will be drawn from deposits in the walls of the arteries, in the same way that a low-calorie diet will drain the body's fat cells. It should be added that most medical authorities doubt that cholesterol buildup in the arteries can be reversed.

Ed Solomon appreciates the occasional absurdity of his new way of life. On dark December mornings, he makes his way along the determinedly curving streets, without sidewalks, laid out by the real estate developers who invented his community. He says, "Around this neighborhood, no one walks anywhere—and here I am, striding along before the sun's even up. One of these days someone's going to call the police about me. If I were walking a dog, of course, I'd be all right, but I've only got a cat, and she won't follow me." Maybe next year, he thinks, he can begin to jog; Pritikin said it was possible. Then he can buy himself a luminous jersey warmup suit and shoes with stripes, and be perfectly acceptable in the suburban landscape.

His diet presents problems. He knows his wife gets tired of making fatless soups for him to take to the office, and sourdough bread—one of his favorite delicacies in the diet, spread with low-fat cottage cheese. After all, she has the boys to cook for, too, and has also been helping tend the tennis courts during the day. When he goes to a restaurant he usually must order spaghetti, specified emphatically without oil or meat sauce, only with tomatoes. But his friends and business associates all know about his angina by now,* and serve him appropriate dishes when he's invited to dinner. Some of them have begun to emulate him. At the office, when the weather is good, a few colleagues go walking with him on the golf course during lunchtime. And he's picked up a small following among people with arteriosclerosis who live in Chicago. Those who have heard he is a Pritikin graduate sometimes call him for advice and encouragement.

Ed can swim again now, though not as strenuously as he used to. "I don't press too hard," he says. "I sort of know how far I can go. I get a little hint from my body, this prenauseous feeling welling up." He feels he can walk endlessly, and at a brisker pace than many healthy people. The stairs from the parking lot to his office have not bothered him for many months.

His general feeling about his angina: "Well, it's there, and I know that it's there. But I can accept it now. My earlier discouragement, the real depression, are gone. I tell myself that I don't have to play tennis every day—or, for that matter, ever. There are plenty of other things to do. All I ask is that I can keep going in the right direction, that this thing doesn't turn around and start getting worse again."

There is something else that Ed thinks about. Growing in

---

* Though he still has not told his mother.

A STRENUOUS MENU

his mind is the possibility that by the time he reaches 50 he may be in a position to change direction in what he does for a living. The tennis club was a beginning, although he acknowledges that the stress of launching it may have had something to do with the onset of angina. Looking back, it seems to him his biggest mistake lay in trying to do everything at once—get the tennis club going, while still holding down a full-time engineering job. Next time he thinks he may give up the engineering and just concentrate on the tennis, "or if not tennis, a skating rink: anything that would be my own."

Just now, however, Ed is trying to decide which of two tennis pros he should hire, and the old engineering outlook has him tied up in indecision: "Two good pros—how do you choose between them? You never know until the guy gets out there and you see how people react to him. It's a matter of judgment. I wake up early and lie in bed thinking about it. I'm a worrier, like my mother."

On the way home from his office after his normal workday is finished, Ed frequently looks in on the tennis club, which is doing a steady business. He stands musing at one side of the vast high room, a windowless, cavern-like space, a remote kind of place. The lights glow downward from above. The occasional cries of the players reverberate briefly, then are swallowed up by the space. The dominant sound is the thump, thump of the tennis balls, a little like a big but erratic heart beating.

．ⅰ　⊹　※

When it comes up against Ed Solomon, health profiling bumps into a problem.

This is because it can deal only in specifics. When it wants to know how much exercise you get, it speaks in terms of numbers of miles walked, or flights of stairs climbed; to get an idea of your nutrition, it asks what you weigh (evidence of your total food intake), and also what your blood levels are for cholesterol and triglycerides (indicating the proportion of animal fats in your diet). These are all measurable factors, with risk percentages well established by medical studies.

But how do you assess the risks of someone who is already sick, as Ed Solomon is with angina? By the severity of his illness? By the treatment he is receiving for it? By his attitude—despairing, hopeful, or somewhere in between? All of these factors must be considered, and a few more besides, many of them almost impossible to express in concrete terms.

Perhaps some day profiling will devise a method for handling this problem. Meanwhile, profile printouts routinely carry a kind of disclaimer (Interhealth's reads: "Pre-existing disease may totally invalidate these results"), and some get more personal. In Ed's case, up near the top of page one of his Interhealth printout are these words:

Note: Some data suggests the following diseases which may significantly increase risk:
Heart disease
Heart disease—angina

Profiling may not be able to measure all of Ed's risks yet, but it does assess something else: his efforts to minimize his illness. Here his printout has nothing but good news. Ed's exercise and diet figures, fed into the computer along with the rest of his data, result in a profile in which, remarkably, current risk and achievable risk are identical for nine of the ten listed causes of death. In other words, in his daily life he has already taken virtually all the steps possible to protect his health and prolong his survival.

Most health profiles carry a fairly long list of suggested ways in which the profilee might reduce risk. Not Ed's. All

A STRENUOUS MENU

you can find on his Interhealth printout is one small entry on page two under Motor Vehicle Accidents: if he were to use a seat belt regularly, he'd lower his risk factor for seat belt usage from 1.0 to .8.

He's working on it.

10
BACK FROM SELF-DESTRUCTION:
Kathleen Mooney, Alcoholic

Early in life Kathleen Mooney began concealing things from other people—things in her life that she couldn't control, or didn't understand. Physical suffering was one. She was afflicted with polio at the age of three and starting at age five underwent a series of operations that dominated her childhood. Much of her time was spent in hospitals; when at home she usually had to wear a cast or a brace, or make her way about on crutches. She was often in pain, but did not allow herself to show it.

She remembers passing other girls on the street and hearing them say, "Oh, there goes a cripple," and she concealed the hurt of that, too.

She formed no friendships with other children. Instead, she worked tremendously hard in the parochial Catholic schools of Sacramento, California, graduating at 16 with honors.

It was at 16, also, that Kathleen had her first drink. Her father mixed it for her. "My father loved good booze, he had that Irish attitude of adoration toward it," she recalls, smiling a little. "It was a Scotch sour he made me, and I remember him kidding around, saying some kind of prayer over it. Then he handed it to me and told me how good I was about to feel. And I did, too; he was absolutely right. From the time I started drinking, it was an instant satisfaction, an immediate psychological tradeoff." By age 18 she had begun to conceal her drinking.

Today Kathleen is 31 and a recovered alcoholic of seven years' standing. She is also a registered nurse whose specialty in psychological counseling allows her to look back on her own life with a trained eye. But what she sees still troubles and saddens her.

She remembers the pivotal year she turned 17, when she entered nursing school. By this time her physical condition was good; her surgery had paid off and she could walk normally, without brace or crutches. The only thing doctors warned her against was being on her feet too much.

If she wasn't supposed to be on her feet, what was she doing in nursing school?

Kathleen smiles a sorrowful smile. "Because I was like that," she says in her soft voice. "Because I wanted challenges. Because at 17 I saw life as one giant challenge, and myself as some kind of superwoman rising up and conquering it. That was how I'd learned to look at things. I wanted to prove that I could do anything I chose, even become a nurse."

She stuck by her resolution, though from the beginning her feet caused her misery. That first year in nursing school she remembers spending whole lunch hours in a bathroom, her feet thrust into the toilet bowl to ease the pain.

She also remembers evenings when she'd go out drinking with some of the other girls. It wasn't long before she realized that she drank differently from them. She always wanted more than they did, and sometimes she drank so much she got sick. This gave her a humiliated feeling, particularly as she did not generally get along well with the other nursing students.

She had never been friendly with people her age and did not know how to be comfortable with them. To make up for this, she tried to impress them with her achievements. In nursing school she pushed herself very hard, not only earning top grades in every subject but in addition, during her second year, becoming editor of the school newspaper.

During that year she also changed her drinking ways. She persuaded the school to convert an unused storeroom into a small private bedroom for herself. There she began keeping scotch in baby food jars, brought back from weekends at home. Now, when she went out with her fellow students, she watched her intake carefully and controlled her behavior; she drank as much as they did, no more. Then she would go back to her room and, alone at last, really drink.

Fresh out of nursing school, Kathleen joined the navy. The year was 1965, and there was a war in Vietnam. She was a drunkard, she says simply, but no one knew it.

At this point she possessed an enormous tolerance for alcohol, and could drink for hours without showing the effects. In boot camp one afternoon, she remembers starting out at four-thirty—Happy Hour, so-called. Someone else who was present kept count. Before she was finished she had consumed 42 vodka gimlets—after which she walked back to barracks.

One expects certain traits in a drinker, but Kathleen does not possess them. She is not a carefree or convivial person. Her soft voice is authoritative, the glance from her blue eyes clear and direct. She is decidedly pretty, with curling brown hair and a happy-looking smile, but even at first meeting what comes across most strongly is an inner seriousness. She is well organized. She is ambitious. It is not surprising that positions of responsibility have always gravitated her way. Typically, the navy after training her made her the nurse in charge of the psychiatric-orthopedics ward at Great Lakes Naval Hospital. She was 20, with very little professional experience of any kind.

Kathleen found the work hard but exciting. The men under her care, she says, "tended to be Green Berets, karate experts—enormous people, many of whom thought they wanted to kill me. Some had been hideously injured, triple amputations, that kind of thing." She often spent eight hours at a stretch changing dressings.

Most of the time she was on her feet, and so she was in constant physical pain. Before long the little toe on her right foot began developing osteomyelitis; eventually it had to be amputated. "To put it plainly, I refused to take care of my feet, and so I lost a toe: that was the message," Kathleen says now. "But I wasn't listening. I kept telling myself I was thriving, that I actually needed all the stress. I was nuts as could be, of course. But on the outside I had this kind of façade I protected myself with—well groomed, professional, kind of a Grace Kelly pose." Though she never drank on the job, she says she would come off duty and sometimes consume a quart of whiskey.

Kathleen says that in women the disease of alcoholism often progresses faster than it does in men, that a man may take fifteen years to arrive at the point of devastation that a woman will reach in five. This seems to have been the case with Kathleen. By the time of her twenty-first birthday, her drinking had begun to make her ill. She started suffering blackouts. She felt out of control and frightened.

Honorably discharged from the navy, she came back to Sacramento, vaguely expecting her family to do something. Her father and mother, her older brother and older sister, all were living at home. Kathleen did not speak of her problem to any of them. Instead, she just drank—"blatantly," she remembers. "I'd come to the kitchen, get out a bottle, set it down on the table, and start to drink. I'd get so drunk I'd fall down and cut my head. Or I'd pass out. And no one said anything. It was just unbelievable. Their denial was acute.

"Years later my mother told me she hadn't realized what was going on. My father said he realized, but didn't know how to handle the problem."

So Kathleen, typically, handled it herself. She handled it by getting married.

His name was Paul and he was a pilot in the navy. The two hoped to help each other: Kathleen informed him beforehand that she was worried about her drinking; he said he'd had serious emotional problems—he'd broken down in his teens and been hospitalized. They decided that love would solve everything. They were married at her parish church in Sacramento.

Three months later they were living in England, and Kathleen was drinking round the clock.

Kathleen describes her two years in England as "a disaster—just catastrophic." She and Paul rented a little cottage out in the countryside. He was in training; she drank.

She remembers taking her two dogs out walking. She wore boots, and into the top of one boot, before setting out, she would slip a pint bottle of brandy. "I still had this crazy idea that I was some kind of lady—the Grace Kelly business again," she says. "For instance, I wouldn't have dreamed of lighting a cigarette on the street." But she'd sneak a drink out of the brandy bottle—after first stepping behind a tree.

Another part of herself, however, was proclaiming the truth to the skies—and just as at home with her family, nothing happened, no one stepped forward to intervene. She began going to a psychiatrist, then dropped him for a second psychiatrist. Neither of them seemed able to grasp

BACK FROM SELF-DESTRUCTION

the simple fact that at 22 she was, in her words, "a raging alcoholic, that that was what was wrong with me, and that I was in the process of destroying myself." They kept suggesting her problem was emotional.

One of them did give her some pills and a notebook, and told her to cut back her drinking by 50 percent. The pills were antidepressants. The notebook was for keeping a record of her drinks. "Well, I tried. At that time I was drinking about 60 drinks every day. Once or twice I brought it down to 40, but I never could get below that. Physiologically, I was just totally addicted.

"My second year in England, I was 23 years old. I was a mess. I weighed 175 pounds. My face was a sort of greenish color. I was so edematous that if I pressed my finger into my skin, I'd leave a dent there that wouldn't go away for an hour. I used to bruise spontaneously—that is, I'd get a bruise on my arm without ever bumping it against anything. This was because my blood was so poisoned. I didn't eat. All I did was drink."

First thing in the morning, before brushing her teeth, Kathleen would start trying to get a drink into her. She'd vomit it up. Then she would try again. She'd keep trying, till finally a drink stayed down. Then she would start facing the day. She knew she would be drinking all day long, but that she would not get high. She was past that point. She explains, "In alcoholism, you reach a stage where liquor quits on you. I mean, the things you used to drink for—the easing of pain, the comfort, the happiness—these things stop coming. But you've got to go on drinking, for negative reasons. You're drinking in order to feel normal. Forget about high, you can't get high no matter how much you drink.

"At this stage I think you become hysterical. My whole life became hysterical. For example, I would argue with Paul, my husband. Then I'd take a whole bottle of antidepressants. We'd go out to dinner, and I would start hallucinating. I'd have to be taken home."

She kept trying to kill herself—"repeatedly—it just seemed the only way out. I'd take pills or stick my head in the oven. Once I drank Sterno, hoping I'd hemorrhage to death." She remembers waking up in an intensive care unit and deliberately ripping away the intravenous feeding tubes. She remembers a spell in a psychiatric hospital. She remembers reporting to some kind of group therapy session falling down drunk.

The strain was too much for Paul. In September of 1969 he suffered a psychotic breakdown and was sent back to the United States for hospitalization. Not long afterward Kathleen also returned. She was met at the airport by her older sister Frances, with whom she was to stay. After two years abroad Kathleen was so physically changed she was almost unrecognizable; her first words were, "If I don't get a bottle of brandy I'm going to die." Within a few short weeks she attempted suicide yet again, and was committed to the psychotic ward of a nearby state hospital.

Though Kathleen did not know it, her life had finally hit bottom. The hospital contained an alcoholism treatment unit. Kathleen was able to get transferred to it, and the following day she enrolled in the hospital's in-patient chapter of Alcoholics Anonymous.

At this point, doctors told her later, her body was so poisoned by alcohol that she could not have continued drinking and stayed alive.

That was eight years ago. Recovering from alcoholism has taken Kathleen Mooney most of those eight years.

The first stage, detoxification or "drying out," occurred within the hospital. Most alcoholics dread detoxification, but Kathleen says cheerfully that hers wasn't so terrible. "It isn't, if you have people around you who understand

BACK FROM SELF-DESTRUCTION

what you're going through, if you can say to them, 'I'm scared; I'm afraid.' " It was that way at the state hospital. She also had a therapist who really helped, a woman who was gentle with her, but who also knew how to be tough when toughness was required. Remembering, Kathleen begins to smile.

"I should explain that although I was a committed patient in a state mental hospital, and a thoroughgoing alcoholic, I still had my little act that I kept up. I wore my hair in a little perfect bun. My makeup was perfect. Having just come from England, I had acquired an English accent. I used to sit there in the hospital with sort of imaginary white gloves on, reading Chaucer, reading the *Iliad* and the *Odyssey*, God knows what—in a state mental hospital! Well, my therapist, she sat down and looked at me, and she said, 'You know, you're full of shit.'

"In the next six weeks, she just broke through that whole veneer; she tore me apart, and let the reality in. I needed it very badly."

On a gray day in early December 1970, Kathleen Mooney, ex-drinker, was released from the hospital. It was a lonely moment. She was permanently separated from her husband. Her parents didn't want her at home. Her only possession of any value was a degree in nursing. She got on a bus and went to Los Angeles. All in one day she found herself both a job and an apartment. She set to work trying to live again.

The first year, Kathleen sometimes says, was the hardest; at other times she says it was the first two years. Whatever the length of the period, it was terribly desolate for her. One day at a time, AA told her, one day meaning twenty-four hours. "Well, sometimes my twenty-four hours went down to five minutes. It was so slow, and it was every day, and it was miserable."

In her comfortable, wood-paneled office Kathleen leans

back and lights another cigarette. What normal people fail to realize, she says, is that an alcoholic isn't just someone who drinks too much. An alcoholic is someone who's gone crazy drinking. And therefore quitting drinking isn't enough. There's still the craziness to deal with.

Ex-drinkers still possess a whole armory of defenses—rationalization, denial, and so forth. They are also extremely impulsive, because with alcohol they have learned to gratify their urges instantly. And their judgments and perceptions are all distorted. "The problems faced by a practicing alcoholic may sound horrendous, but really they're sort of limited. Like: *If I go to such and such a place, will I be able to get enough to drink?* Or: *Shall I drink Scotch, or save it for tomorrow morning and have vodka today?* These are the kinds of decisions an alcoholic worries about. When you get out into the real world, without any bottle, you discover you're just infantile, you don't know what to do about anything."

Worst of all, though, Kathleen says, alcoholics lose their capacity to relate to other people. "No matter who comes into your life, when you're an alcoholic you're going to be interested in people on just one basis: Will they be a vehicle—or an impediment? Will they make it easier for you to drink—or will they make it harder? That's your sole concern. And I don't care if it's booze, or heroin, or Valium—if you're sneaking it, you can't relate honestly to any other human being. You can't relate honestly to yourself."

Kathleen's problem was compounded because she hadn't known as a child how to relate to other children. Now in social situations she felt clumsy, self-conscious, irrationally frightened—"like one big, huge sore thumb." This was true even at AA meetings which, she recalls, "scared the bejesus out of me." But she made herself keep going. "I knew I had to, had to force myself through this slow process day after day, of just trying to crack a little of the cement I'd built up around me. It was the hardest experience of my life, it went far beyond any other pain I went through, this longing to belong, if only to AA. To me, it meant belonging to the human race." During that first year, Kathleen attended an AA meeting every day.

Kathleen did not drink again, but many problems arose in her life, and almost all of them were alcohol-related, she now recognizes. One of the most frightening occurred in her first month in Los Angeles. At the hospital where she found work, she began having trouble with her feet again. She wasn't drinking, she was alone, she was frequently miserable. She began taking Darvon for the pain. "One pill every six to eight hours," she remembers. "Well, inside of three weeks I was taking 32 a day. By the handful. The handful! Anything to put in my mouth to make me feel better!

"It's a terrifying thing to realize—that you're out of control not just with liquor, but with virtually anything you put into your mouth. And suddenly I saw the danger I was in."

AA had assigned Kathleen a sponsor, someone for her to telephone if she felt she needed to drink, and now, after several days' hesitation, Kathleen called her for the first time. In retrospect she sees this as a major step in her recovery. "You can't solve these things by yourself," she says. "You've got to be able to say to another human being, 'I'm gobbling down Darvon, and I don't know what to do.' " After the episode with the Darvon, Kathleen found herself calling someone in AA almost every day.

Nevertheless, it was three years before she learned to feel comfortable at AA meetings. She says that the ability to care for other people came very slowly to her. "I think that first I had to learn to care for myself, and this happened only in stages. My feet, for example. It was in 1972, two years after I stopped drinking, that it finally dawned on me—I was crazy trying to work as a nurse! Well, I went back to school and earned a degree in psychology. After that I was an R.N. with a B.A., I didn't have to be on my feet all day any more."

But other problems persisted. Repeatedly, she found herself taking on too many challenges, plunging into impossible situations without looking first. During this period, when she was back in school getting her degree, she met a man in AA and moved into his house with him. He had five children, but that didn't deter her. "I just made up my mind I wanted to live with this man, take care of the kids, carry 21 credits at school, and work full time. And I did it. I'd come home from school, cook dinner for seven people, feed the dog, wash the clothes, deal with the kids. For a year and a half!"

Throughout her recovery Kathleen also suffered from money problems. She had a charge card at Bullock's. Wandering around the store, she would come across a $45 planter that caught her fancy; never mind the price tag—if she liked it, she bought it. She'd purchase whole sets of bathroom linen, expensive clothes for herself, gifts for the children, all on impulse. "It's what psychoanalysts call oral," she says. "It's as though you've got to get something into yourself very quickly, right away; you can't stop and think it over rationally.

"And it's so much like drinking. I mean, when you go out and splurge on a credit card, you love the hell out of it while you're doing it. Then two days later the remorse is unbelievable. You look around at all the junk you bought: *Why did I do it! What's the matter with me!*"

In 1975, five years after she stopped drinking, Kathleen was still constantly in debt. That year she began going to a psychotherapist who, as a condition of treatment, agreed to see her each session only for the length of time she could pay for on the spot, in cash. Often, at first, this meant she got only fifteen minutes with him. But ultimately she was able to pay off her debts and tear up the credit cards.

Therapy also helped Kathleen to understand her life, to trace the subtle connections between her pain-filled childhood and the violent alcoholism of her early twenties, and back to her childhood again. "I had eight major operations in ten years," she says. "Starting at age 5. This was my life."

She remembers being wheeled into operating rooms, where people in strange clothes wore masks over their faces, and no one explained anything to her.

She remembers church. "I used to pray to God to let me know what I had done," she says. "I remember going to church and trying to pray. I had become a cripple when I was 3 years old, after all. There had to be some reason. After confession, the angels were supposed to come down and clean up your soul. But it never happened to me. My soul stayed black; I visualized it."

She also has very early memories of her father. "Sometimes I'd find him looking at me, and I'd know that if I showed distress he was going to break down. So I'd start performing. Sometimes I dreaded having to do it. But I did it.

"No one ever saw me in pain as a child; I *never* complained of it. A nurse might anticipate, might come round with an injection. But I never asked for help with pain, never. I never cried."

The only time that her control used to slip was just before an operation, when the stretcher was brought to her room. "I was all right till I got on the stretcher. Then I would start shaking and wouldn't be able to stop. No matter what my mind told my body, my body just went on shaking. I finally asked my parents not to be present at those moments."

The adults around Kathleen praised her fortitude. But

she feels that they also, in a way, came to count on it, it so eased their own role. She says, "They were armed against my complaining, even though I never did complain. I remember the nuns saying to me, 'Aren't you glad you've got this cross to bear, so you can have your purgatory here on earth?' " She also recalls a minor incident in her teens when, on her way to school, she knocked her foot against a curb and could hardly walk afterward. For once, she did complain—and was rebuffed. "My mother didn't believe me, she thought I was trying to get out of going to school. Then one of the nuns came up; do you know what she said? 'I wept because I had no shoes, until I saw a man who had no feet.' She threw *that* at me!"

Today Kathleen understands the self-destructive side of her childhood stoicism. She says firmly, "I should have screamed and cried when I was in pain, like anyone else. I should have learned to reach out to human beings." Therapy, she says, has helped her understand these things.

But her actual recovery she credits to Alcoholics Anonymous. At AA Kathleen learned the nature of her disease, and how not to drink in different situations. More important, she met people who had once been as hopelessly alcoholic as herself, and who nevertheless had recovered. As she became familiar with their stories, she slowly began to identify with their recovery.

"There's a lot of spirituality in AA—go to a meeting and you can't help but pick it up," Kathleen says. She believes this spirituality is important and that it works, even with a person like herself who is not very religious. She begins outlining the well known "twelve steps" of AA:

"In step 1, you admit that you've become powerless over alcohol—which in most cases is pretty obvious. Then it starts getting harder. In step 2 you say that only a higher power can restore you to sanity; and in the third step, you resolve to turn your life and will over to this higher power.

BACK FROM SELF-DESTRUCTION

In step 4 you take moral inventory of yourself, and in step 5 you share it with another person. And so on." Taken all together, Kathleen says, the twelve steps comprise a kind of exercise in humility and are therefore highly therapeutic; ironically, most alcoholics are filled with pride—"pride and grandiosity; they'll sit there drunk as skunks, all the time proclaiming how wonderful they are!"

Kathleen says that step 3—"turning my life over"— "was the crucial point for me. It means you have to stop trying to control everything, stop manipulating people and situations in your life. The message is: 'Sweetie, you've been doing things your way for a long while and you've gotten nowhere but in a drug tank, or in jail, or in a mental hospital; you've lost your life. Now move over a little.'

"It was the hardest thing in the world for me to do, but I was finally able to do it, and it has given me a great deal of comfort. For me, I think, God happens to be just the power of things outside me. I have no control over this power whatsoever. Nevertheless, I know that if I do good things, for myself and for other people, then good things will be given back to me. This is a happy feeling, a serenity, a kind of faith. I'm not lonely."

Today Kathleen runs a Troubled Employee Program for a large industrial corporation in Los Angeles. "Our key word is 'stress,' " she says, "the kind of situations that send people into mental breakdown, alcoholism, or drugs." She says that alcoholism is a major problem in industry, sometimes overt, sometimes concealed by cross-addiction. Women in particular, she says, become cross-addicted— "You know, they'll carry a bottle of Valium in their purse and take six or seven during the day. That keeps them going till nighttime, when they return home and cross back to drinking again."

Not long ago Kathleen began a private practice in therapy on a small scale, at the invitation of a Los Angeles psychiatrist who knew about her background and wanted her in his office. Announcements were sent out and a small party was given. One of the people who showed up was Kathleen's old therapist from the state hospital. "I always used to call her around Thanksgiving time to let her know I was okay. Now, lo and behold, she came to my open house. She brought me a single red rose. She said, 'Having been part of your recovery has made my career complete.' I can't tell you how that made me feel."

Full-time job, part-time private practice—and Kathleen is also, just now, back at school, working for a master's degree in psychology at UCLA. Is she headed toward trouble again, taking on too much?

She smiles, but on the whole thinks not. "Oh I still hit the ceiling sometimes," she admits. "I get this itchy feeling, give me a challenge, send me to Bimini to start something, here's the tools, go do it—and I'd love it. I'd love it. But I'm not doing it. I'm not even trying for a Ph.D. The M.A.'s going to be enough for me."

Not long ago she re-signed the lease on her apartment—one of the nicest moments in her recovery, she says. "Till now I never stayed in one spot longer than two years, and I *never* re-signed a lease. It's just amazing to me, the stability this makes me feel." There is silence as Kathleen surveys her future. Then, "The biggest challenge in *my* life is to be good to myself; that's probably the hardest responsibility I'll ever have," says Kathleen Mooney pleasantly, rising to end the conversation.

* * *

On standard health profiles the dividing line between heavy social drinking and alcoholism is set at 40 drinks per week, a figure that can't help but bring a smile to Kathleen's face. "Forty drinks! That's a drop in the bucket to a real alcoholic," she says. At the height of her drinking career she often consumed 60 drinks per *day*—in other words, about ten times the health profile figure.

The professionals in profiling have their reasons, however. First of all, they point out, the actual designation used is "40 drinks *or more* per week." Second, while it is possible to quibble over the meaning of the word "alcoholic," one plain fact remains: Anyone consuming over 40 drinks weekly already has a serious drinking problem which measurably affects his or her health prospects.

Kathleen reached the 40-drinks-per-week level at the age of 18, during her second year in nursing school. Would a health profile at that time have shocked her into self-recognition, spurring her to change the course of her life and perhaps averting the calamities that lay just ahead? No one can answer for sure, but it is possible to look back today and construct a retrospective profile based on the facts and figures of Kathleen's eighteenth year. The result is a strong, clear, perhaps even sobering, document. The highlights:

- At age 18, Kathleen's overall risk of death was more than three times the average for her age, race, and sex.
- Her risk age was *21 years* greater than her chronological age, making her the equivalent, healthwise, of a woman of 39.
- In the decade to come, her three likeliest causes of death were all violent: motor vehicle accidents, suicide, and homicide.*

An unappealing prospect, in short. Here is Kathleen's retrospective profile in detail:

* Because it takes years to develop, cirrhosis of the liver doesn't even appear on Kathleen's list of risks at age 18; on her accompanying age-40 projection, however, it occupies first place, with a risk of death ten times the average.

HEALTH RISK PROFILE

Kathleen Mooney, age 18, white.

Age in terms of present health, 39.

Achievable health age, 25.

An average white woman your age has 600 chances per 100,000 of dying in the next ten years; your risks are 209% greater than the average. You can, however, reduce these risks by 62%.

FACTORS OFFERING THE GREATEST REDUCTION IN RISK:	THE NUMBER OF YEARS TO BE GAINED BY ALTERING THOSE FACTORS:
Drinking	11.0 years
Smoking	1.7 years
Other factors	1.3 years
Total	14.0 years

Your risks of death within the next ten years in descending importance:

1. MOTOR VEHICLE ACCIDENTS

AVERAGE RISK	197 ●●●●●●●●●●
YOUR CURRENT RISK	1,202 ●●●●●●●●●●●●●●●●●●●● ●●●●●●●●●●●●●●●●●●●● ●●●●●●●●●●●●●●●●●●●●
YOUR ACHIEVABLE RISK	276 ●●●●●●●●●●●●●●

INDICATORS OF RISK	RISK RATING	WAYS TO REDUCE RISK	RISK RATING
Alcohol consumption—40 drinks per week or more	5.0	No drinks before driving	.5
Mileage—25,000 yearly as driver or passenger	2.0		
Seat belt use—less than 10% of time	1.1	Use seat belts always	.8

BACK FROM SELF-DESTRUCTION

2. SUICIDE

AVERAGE RISK	52 ●●●●●●●●●●
YOUR CURRENT RISK	208 ●●
YOUR ACHIEVABLE RISK	78 ●●●●●●●●●●●●●●●

INDICATORS OF RISK	RISK RATING	WAYS TO REDUCE RISK	RISK RATING
Depression—yes	2.5	Seeking help	1.5
Family history of suicide—none	1.0		
Alcohol consumption—40 drinks per week or more	2.5	Not drinking	1.0

3. HOMICIDE

AVERAGE RISK	40 ●●●●●●●●●●
YOUR CURRENT RISK	100 ●●●●●●●●●●●●●●●●●●●●●●●●●
YOUR ACHIEVABLE RISK	40 ●●●●●●●●●●

INDICATORS OF RISK	RISK RATING	WAYS TO REDUCE RISK	RISK RATING
No arrests for violence	1.0		
Does not carry weapon	1.0		
Alcohol consumption—40 drinks per week or more	2.5	Not drinking	1.0

4. PNEUMONIA

AVERAGE RISK	13 ●●●●●●●●●●
YOUR CURRENT RISK	42 ●●●●●●●●●●●●●●●●●●●●●●●●●●●●●●●●
YOUR ACHIEVABLE RISK	13 ●●●●●●●●●●

THE LONGEVITY FACTOR

INDICATORS OF RISK	RISK RATING	WAYS TO REDUCE RISK	RISK RATING
Alcohol consumption—40 drinks per week or more	3.0	6 drinks or less weekly	1.0
No history of bacterial pneumonia	1.0		
No history of emphysema	1.0		
Smoker—1½ packs per day	1.2	Not smoking	1.0

5. POISONINGS

AVERAGE RISK	17 ••••••••••
YOUR CURRENT RISK	17 ••••••••••
YOUR ACHIEVABLE RISK	17 ••••••••••

No risk indicators have been established for this cause of death.

6. LEUKEMIA AND ALEUKEMIA

AVERAGE RISK	17 ••••••••••
YOUR CURRENT RISK	17 ••••••••••
YOUR ACHIEVABLE RISK	17 ••••••••••

No risk indicators have been established for this cause of death.

7. STROKE

AVERAGE RISK	13 ••••••••••
YOUR CURRENT RISK	17 ••••••••••••••
YOUR ACHIEVABLE RISK	10 ••••••••

INDICATORS OF RISK	RISK RATING	WAYS TO REDUCE RISK	RISK RATING
Current blood pressure 135/80	.8		
Current cholesterol—not given, average used	1.0		

BACK FROM SELF-DESTRUCTION

INDICATORS OF RISK	RISK RATING	WAYS TO REDUCE RISK	RISK RATING
Diabetes—none	1.0		
Smoker—1½ packs per day	1.5	Not smoking	1.0
History of abnormal electrocardiogram—none	1.0		

8. CONGENITAL CIRCULATORY DEFECTS

AVERAGE RISK	11 ●●●●●●●●●●
YOUR CURRENT RISK	11 ●●●●●●●●●●
YOUR ACHIEVABLE RISK	11 ●●●●●●●●●●

No risk indicators have been established for this cause of death.

9. BRAIN CANCER OR CANCER OF CENTRAL NERVOUS SYSTEM

AVERAGE RISK	9 ●●●●●●●●●●
YOUR CURRENT RISK	9 ●●●●●●●●●●
YOUR ACHIEVABLE RISK	9 ●●●●●●●●●●

No risk indicators have been established for this cause of death.

10. DROWNINGS

AVERAGE RISK	8 ●●●●●●●●●●
YOUR CURRENT RISK	8 ●●●●●●●●●●
YOUR ACHIEVABLE RISK	8 ●●●●●●●●●●

No risk indicators have been established for this cause of death.

OTHER

Your risk of death from all other causes in the next ten years totals 223 out of 100,000.

11

CHANGING ACROSS THE BOARD:
Jack Kodaly, "Normal" Health

Jack Kodaly of San Francisco is well over six feet tall, with sandy hair graying slightly at the sideburns, wide shoulders, long legs, and a very pleasant and easy manner. Handsome and strong and kind, he makes you think of a good guy out of some children's Western. Actually, he is a line member on San Francisco's respected fire department force. Over a period of twenty-three years he has worked his way up to captain; he has been decorated a number of times.

Fighting fires is highly physical work. Firemen have to be able to run up sixteen flights of stairs while pulling heavy hoses behind them, chop their way through smoldering walls, and heft victims down ladders. "One way or another we're all physical fitness nuts—the job demands it," Jack says. Even the schedule is extreme: the forty-eight hours he works per week are packed into two twenty-four-hour shifts, leaving the rest of his time completely free. This is not as relaxing as it sounds.

Five years ago the Institute of Health Research at the University of California invited the members of the city fire department to participate in a study it was making, among healthy people, of individual fluctuations in cholesterol, blood pressure, and other physiological measurements of body chemistry. Along with several fellow firemen Jack decided to investigate, though he wasn't particularly worried about his health at the time. "I knew I was basically strong and capable," he remembers. This confidence was backed up, on the whole, by the examination that the Institute performed on him. His cholesterol rating was 253 and his blood pressure 145/86, both considered within normal limits by most physicians for a man of 43. Dr. George Williams, director of the Institute, however, believes that *normal* is not synonymous with *healthy*. He persuaded Jack to join the Institute's program. This would involve going to work on three areas of his life: diet, exercise, and smoking. Then periodically he would report back to the Institute for retesting—to discover just what effect his efforts were having on his body chemistry.

Kodaly entered the program with many assets, among them good heredity and upbringing. There has been heart disease in his family but most of his forebears lived long, full lives before it struck. His paternal grandfather came to the United States from the Austro-Hungarian Empire, settled in the Dakotas when that area was still a Territory, and became a successful farmer. "He was an iron man," Jack says. "He signed his name with an X, but he knew how to make a buck; he held fifty or sixty mortgages. He lived to be 88 or 89." Equally sturdy was the stock on his mother's side: his maternal grandmother, Russian-born, survived well into her nineties before her heart gave out.

Jack grew up in the tough Mission section of San Francisco, where he learned early to take care of himself. Starting at age 7 or 8, he helped support the family. "After school I shined shoes, washed dishes, worked as plasterer's helper, longshoreman, hod-carrier. I remember cleaning two hundred chickens for a butcher one time." He was also a street fighter who never lost a fight after the age of 12. In 1950 he was drafted and sent to Korea, where he fought in the line for eight months and twenty days, was wounded twice, and was awarded the Silver Star.

Food was taken seriously in the Kodaly family, partly for religious reasons. When his maternal grandparents emigrated from Russia, they brought with them their faith in a wing of the Russian Orthodox Church known as the Milk Drinkers. The Milk Drinkers ate a lot of vegetables and sour cream. They usually boiled their meat, avoiding any with a high fat content such as pork. They did not smoke or drink alcohol. Jack remembers escorting his grandmother at eight o'clock some Sunday mornings to her church on the top of Russian Hill and being told to call for her again at five o'clock. "I asked her what she would do all that time. 'Oh,' she said, 'we pray, we cry, we laugh—we have an awfully good time.' " The Milk Drinkers ate at a long table in the church. The women set out tomatoes and cucumbers, never peeling them. They thought they lost all their food value when they were peeled.

In his home, as a child, Jack remembers tomatoes bought by the case, huge bags of peaches and oranges. Candy, considered a poison, was forbidden, "and if you drank a Coke you got slugged." He also consumed lavish quantities of milk—"a gallon a day, I'll bet." He was an infantryman in Korea before he got his first dental cavity.

In adulthood, Jack continued the eating patterns he'd learned as a child, confident they could do him nothing but good. Eggs, for instance. A bachelor who cooked his own meals, he might prepare himself a three-egg omelet for a bedtime snack, then get up the next morning and have four eggs for breakfast; often he ate nine eggs in a single day. It wasn't until he joined the IHR program that he learned how this diet, continued, could inflate his cholesterol count. There were other surprises as well. All his life Jack had been adding salt to everything that entered his mouth, even packaged potato chips. Now he learned that salt can help to cause high blood pressure.

Armed with Dr. Williams' admonitions plus a copy of the American Heart Association's diet recommendations, Kodaly went home to alter his habits.

Many of the changes proved easy for him. He had always liked fish, poultry, and veal, and found it no hardship to limit his beef intake to twice a week (down from twice a day). Going without salt was difficult, but his consumption of eggs swiftly dropped to two or three a week, butter to a quarter pound a month.

The physical exercise which Williams recommended was no imposition either, because Jack, a high school athlete, had always liked to run. In the army he remembers having to run four miles during basic training, wearing a full pack and helmet, and he always felt exuberant afterward. Out of the army and back in San Francisco, he continued running once in a while, usually at the beach.

Jack worked out a plan to run on a regular basis: two or three miles through Golden Gate Park each time he had a day off.

What was anguish for Kodaly, however, was to give up his 2½ packs of cigarettes a day. He had tried before, repeatedly, always without success. "Most of the things I've wanted to do in my life, I've had the self-discipline for," he says now. "But I found cigarettes a terrible enemy. I used them to wake up in the morning and to go to sleep at night, when I was standing up and when I was sitting down. I'd come out of a building after a fire, coughing and spitting from the smoke, and the first thing I wanted was a cigarette." Back in 1953, when he joined the fire department, virtually all the firemen he knew also smoked. But by the early seventies many had quit. Jack wanted desperately to join them.

For six long months he struggled with the problem, using tricks out of pamphlets, any device he could think of. He tried keeping the cigarettes in his car, to make smoking inconvenient. When he did light a cigarette, he'd force himself to put it out again after one or two puffs. He'd wake in the morning and see how long he could go before lighting up, extending the time of deprivation each morning: first until after he'd had coffee; then till he was on his way to work; then till after roll call. Pretty soon he'd reached the point where he could survive without smoking until ten in the morning. But he was still smoking.

Vacation loomed. He made up his mind that this year he would devote his four weeks off exclusively to becoming an ex-smoker.

The tensions were terrible. "I'll bet you couldn't have driven a nail into the side of my neck," he says. At night he woke every three or four hours, longing for cigarettes. He had to give up coffee in the morning because it roused such cravings.

One of the few things that helped was sunflower seeds, which he says he ate "by the ton. I ate so many, my lips split from the salt. After that I bought them unsalted. Unshelled, too—otherwise you'd eat them so fast you'd be sick. And you need that click, click, click of getting the shell off. But the shells were everywhere, in my pockets, in the car, under the chairs, in bed."

Three-quarters of the way through his vacation, Kodaly reported at IHR for a testing appointment, and told the staff there what he had been going through. They gave him advice and encouragement, and he went back home with his determination bolstered. By now he was down to one or two cigarettes a day.

As it turned out, the worst was over. Back at work, Jack made the happy discovery that the roster at the Chinatown stationhouse where he was now assigned contained not one cigarette smoker. A few days later, for the first time, he got through an entire twenty-four hours without a cigarette. He felt elated. He was on his way.

With each day that passed his confidence grew, and gradually he stopped thinking of cigarettes. "You know what was a nice moment?" he recalls. "I was walking around one night when I got the urge to smoke. And suddenly I realized I hadn't thought of smoking all day long. Here it was, eleven o'clock at night!"

He also began to feel very good physically, so brimming with energy that he had to find some way of expending it; at this point he started running in earnest in Golden Gate Park.

His sense of well-being was not illusion but physiological fact, as was demonstrated periodically by his tests for pulmonary capacity, heart rate, and blood pressure at IHR, particularly the pulmonary measure. Well into his exercise program, and a year after his last cigarette, Kodaly received in the mail one day a memo from one Institute doctor to another commenting on the dramatic changes that had taken place in his pulmonary function. "Fascinating, remarkable, almost unbelievable" were the words used.

Jack read the memo. Then he hurried off to the grocery store, filled up a bag with prosciutto, Fontina cheese, and other delicacies, and drove over to the Institute where, jubilant and grateful, he threw a small party for the staff.

Since joining the IHR program five years ago, Kodaly has lost 30 pounds, to 176, and taken in his belt four notches. His cholesterol count is down to 191, his resting pulse to 60 beats a minute, and his blood pressure is 116 over 62. He is happy with both his diet and his exercise program, but hardly fanatical about either. In the firehouse the men take turns cooking, so except when Jack himself is in charge, not all the meals conform to Heart Association standards by any means. This doesn't upset him. "If they happen to have corned beef I just take a small helping, and maybe pop down to the store for some fruit later," he says. "But actually I can't remember having corned beef in over a year now. People have changed—within the fire department you can see it. Practically everyone is aware of cholesterol and salt now."

The same is true of exercise. In the middle of the night, driving back to the stationhouse after a fire, Kodaly often sees runners on the dark streets of his city. "It's three or four o'clock in the morning, and they'll be jogging along the Embarcadero." He also knows more than a few firemen who run fifteen or twenty miles at a stretch, three times a week. Jack runs strictly by daylight, in modest two- to four-mile snatches, at a speed of about nine miles an hour.

Once in a while he even smokes a cigarette, then swiftly returns to abstention. His worst lapse occurred two years ago when his stationhouse got a call about an 18-year-old youth who was out on a ledge of the twenty-fifth floor of an office building, threatening to jump. Shortly, Jack was on the ledge with him, hoping to talk him out of it. The boy had a knife. Not far away, just out of sight, other firemen stood by anxiously with ropes, but Jack couldn't carry one himself. "If you bring a rope, that spooks a jumper."

Jack tells the story. "He'd say, 'Well, this is it,' and begin to move. I'd say, 'No, wait, have a cigarette.' I'd light up two and give him one, and we'd smoke together. I ended up smoking several packs of cigarettes. But it worked. It kept him from jumping." At one point, the two also ate hamburgers and shared a beer. Altogether, six hours passed before Jack saw his chance and was able to overpower the boy and bring him to safety. "He was sick in the head. It was really sad," Jack says.

The San Francisco fire department gets many suicide cases. It doesn't succeed in preventing all of them.

As for himself, after the episode on the twenty-fifth floor ledge, Jack went on a smoking spree that lasted two weeks. Then he quit again, quietly this time.

Though he says he is happier than he's ever been, Kodaly sometimes wonders if he wants to remain a fireman forever. He could retire soon, and there are times when he thinks of going back to school. After he got out of the army he took night courses; in fact, he first joined the fire department because of all the time off, which he planned to spend studying—during that period he hoped to become a labor lawyer. "I've never cared for uniforms," he muses, "but I've spent my life in them. How about that."

In addition, the easygoing side of his nature yearns for a more relaxed way of life. "I enjoy talking. I enjoy food, I enjoy trees, I love a million things. Sometimes I think of the old Italian *bocce* players I see at North Beach. They know how to live. A good wife, a good meal, a little sunshine. What more does anyone need?"

But underneath the geniality lie other qualities. Jack did not care for his eight months in Korea, but they taught him a lot and he speaks of them often. He remembers the danger, the frigid weather, the terrible food.

He also remembers the men with whom he served. "A third were maybe average, and a third were really burdens. But I'd say the other third were just excellent—quietly tough men.

"At the time I went to Korea, our troops had just taken a bad beating. There were seven or eight planeloads flown from here—and seven hours later we were in the middle of it. It's a little hard to explain, but when that happens, the fear just leaves you. I think you're too taken up with practical problems—should you go around this rock, or that one? You're so involved you're not afraid."

This kind of involvement is what enables a fireman to plunge into a flaming building, to coax a would-be suicide away from a twenty-fifth floor ledge—or to rescue an injured man trapped in his car following an automobile accident, as Jack did on one recent night. "The guy was pinned in his Volkswagen, hysterical. And we had to cut him out, while he was screaming and bleeding. It was tough, I'll tell you. You know, we were concerned about him, and it wasn't easy getting the metal off him, and he was pinned good; so we were doing this very difficult physical thing, and all the time taking the stress of it, too." Jack fell silent for a moment. Then he said, "We got him out, though. He's going to be okay."

At times his station gets calls to rescue animals too, just like the firemen in comic strips.

"It's a rewarding experience to save a life, human or animal," Jack Kodaly says simply.

* * *

The Institute of Health Research, which helped Jack Kodaly mend his ways, does not employ a predictive health profile, but its program resembles profiling in that it takes certain accepted physiological measurements of health—blood pressure, cholesterol levels, and the like—and in effect sets standards toward which people can work. Thus six months after Jack changed his eating patterns, he learned through an IHR visit that his cholesterol level had dropped substantially. This encouraged him to continue his efforts, and a year later it had dropped further still.

A major purpose of both systems is to help people *want* to change, by rating them in terms as concrete as the scores in a basketball game. Health profiling, however, does this by comparing your statistics with those of hundreds of thousands of other Americans, while the IHR program compares you chiefly to yourself—to the baseline figures established as normal for you as an individual, during the first phase of early tests. Approximately thirty different health factors are measured.

Dr. George Williams, head of IHR, suspects these baseline figures are extremely important. He isn't just trying to influence people, he's also investigating a theory—namely, that what constitutes "normal" is a highly individual matter, and that ratings from blood tests that would be healthy in one person may signal the advent of disease in another. If this proves to be so, then careful tracking might establish a kind of early warning system that could become an important breakthrough in the practice of preventive medicine.

Meanwhile, IHR's program of repeated testing helps people to change, because it confirms their efforts with concrete and objective ratings. Here is Kodaly's record during his first 18 months in the program, in terms of blood cholesterol and blood triglycerides (both have been implicated in heart disease):

	ON ENTERING THE PROGRAM (DECEMBER 1973)	6 MONTHS LATER (JUNE 1974)	12 MONTHS AFTER THAT (JUNE 1975)
Cholesterol	253.5	197	191
Triglycerides	165.75	154	107

During the same period his weight fell from 205 to 185, and his blood pressure from 145/86 to 122/68. But the most striking change was respiratory: in 12 months Jack's pulmonary diffusion capacity, to name just one measurement, rose from 24.0 to 40.1, startling even his lung specialist, Dr. Robert J. Fallat, who hurried back to his files to re-check the figures. But no errors were found, and all of the results had been corroborated by either duplicate or triplicate testing.

"Jack Kodaly is an interesting case," Dr. Fallat says. "Why did his lung capacity improve so dramatically? I'm pretty certain it's not because he stopped smoking—if that were the reason, the changes would have shown up earlier, in the first couple of months. Because he runs? But the general consensus is that exercise won't improve lung function to any very major extent.

"The chief benefits of running are considered to be cardiovascular, not pulmonary, you see. Maybe this premise needs to be looked at more carefully."

12
OUTRANGING THE AGE TABLES:
Emily Eastman, 85

Not all people fit into the health profile system. Miss Emily Eastman of New York City is 85 years old, well past the limits of the Geller-Steele age tables. Yet it is worth tracing her story to learn some of the ways in which another quality affects health. That quality is attitude.

Miss Eastman speaks in a British–New York accent, with vigor, wit, and velocity. The accent is valid; born to an American father and an English mother in London in 1892, and brought to this country when she was 3, she has over the years made numerous visits back to England. Her longest consecutive stay was in London during the German bombing from 1940 through 1942. "It was not courageous on my part. I just thought I'd rather be there than here," is her point of view.

Miss Eastman is tall and handsome, though slightly bent at the shoulders, but she dismisses that too: "It's not the kind of arthritis that's painful—doesn't bother me a bit." Her white hair is cut short and combed casually. She still has good legs, and shows them off with graceful shoes.

"My health is excellent, absolutely excellent," says Miss

THE LONGEVITY FACTOR

Eastman. "The doctor laughs. He says, 'How are you?' and I say, 'I'm fine.' I really truly mean I haven't an ache or a pain. I have two eyes, two lips, two ears that work perfectly, in short I'm as healthy today as I was thirty years ago. I don't stand up in buses quite as well, that's true—I wobble a bit, my balance is slightly off.

"The only real illness I've had is cancer. I've had two mastectomies."

Miss Eastman's narrative:

"The first time was in '63. I had booked a berth on the *Queen Mary* to attend a wedding in Sussex, and I had to get a new vaccination. The doctor said, 'So long as you're here, let's look you over.' And he put me on my back and poked around and found this little lump deep down in my breast. He said it had to be operated on, but if everything went all right I could convalesce on the ship, on my way to the wedding.

"However, things did *not* go all right, the beastly thing wouldn't *heal*. I had to have a skin graft. I was in the hospital exactly four weeks, and missed the wedding completely.

"After that I went sailing along perfectly until 1973, when I had a fall getting out of an elevator in London, and I wrenched my back. It remained painful even after I returned to New York.

"My surgeon, Dr. Powers, had an office right in back of Bloomingdale's, so one day I dropped in to ask him what to do. He said the same thing as the previous doctor: 'Now that you're here, let's look you over.' He found that my nipple was turned in, apparently sometimes a sign of cancer. He took me to a mirror.

" 'Hadn't you noticed?' he asked, and I answered, 'I don't put on my glasses when I take a bath.' Well, I don't, you know.

"That time there was absolutely no trouble, I was out in about ten days. Didn't bother me at all."

Says a nephew of Miss Eastman, a 60-year-old physician practicing in Atlanta, "The truth is that Aunt Emily is going a heck of a lot stronger than I am myself. I'm convinced she simply rose above her two malignancies.

"Did she tell you," he adds, "that she developed postoperative atelectasis—collapse of the lung—after the first mastectomy, but ten days after she left the hospital she was off to visit her English relatives?"

Most people do not rise above cancer. Why Aunt Emily? Perhaps it has to do with her general health, which in turn has to do with her upbringing.

Miss Eastman doesn't gain weight, because she eats plenty of fruits and vegetables, just as she was brought up to do. She's always walked a lot, and therefore needs no special exercise program. She consumes only one cigarette a day, so why stop smoking?

She seldom thinks about her health, but will do so on request.

She recalls the meals in her childhood home. "I remember the dining room chairs, oak, with leather seats. We'd sit there at breakfast, our chins just coming up over the table, poking away at an orange with our spoons. My father used to have chops and creamed potatoes for breakfast; but we always had oatmeal, and the orange. We had dinner in the middle of the day until we were 14, while the mothers and fathers ate at night, fancy things, squabs and whatnot. We would have tea at five o'clock, then sandwiches for the evening meal.

"We were very carefully fed, extraordinarily so, I think. And we had to go to bed at very precise hours, and were just plain brought up. Children were, in those days."

Miss Eastman's father, born in 1839, was a stock broker in New York. One morning in 1907, on his way down to Wall Street, he was knocked down by a trolley on Sixth Avenue and killed, leaving the upbringing of the family to his wife. Just after the end of World War I the mother herself was diagnosed as having pernicious anemia, then considered incurable, so Emily closed the home in which they had been living and, taking along Alice, the English maid, rented a small house for the three of them in rural Connecticut. Emily's sisters and brothers were married by then, and away from home.

Emily remembers this as perhaps the happiest period of her life. She was twenty-five years old, and had been restless and bored for several years. "In those days you weren't expected to do anything but sit around, waiting to get married. And I didn't *get* married. In Connecticut, however, I had a job to do, the house, the whole show. I was very congenial with my mother. We moved her into a room that looked over a lovely valley up to the Berkshires." They lived there for five years, until 1923, when her mother, despite many transfusions, finally died. Emily, 31, inherited a small income, enough for one person to live on, and her family and friends all demanded, "What are you going to do with your life?"

Emily first moved to an apartment in New York, with Alice, and took up her mother's interest in an old ladies' home run by the Episcopal Church. "Mother had been a trustee of the institution, and I kind of inherited that from her. I found that I liked it very much. I liked the old ladies." Emily spent a year in New York, then made a trip to England to arrange retirement for Alice and to visit relatives and friends. One morning in 1925, while doing her hair, she had a sudden idea: She would enroll at Cambridge.

Her year at Cambridge, she says, was wonderful. "It came at the end of a period of strain, what with my mother's death, and was great fun for me. I bought an old car, and got to know a young Irishman who loved driving. One day after the term was finished, and all the examinations were over with, we went off for a day in the countryside. On the way home, suddenly, the car collapsed. Finally we got somebody to fix it, but the upshot was that it was about three in the morning when we got back to Cambridge, speeding at all of 30 miles an hour on the empty roads. I remember to this day, I had this absolutely glorious knowledge that there was nobody in the entire *world* who knew where I was. That glorious feeling of complete and total *freedom*."

It was something she was never to lose, although family ties—and her old ladies—soon pulled her back to the United States. Nieces and nephews were beginning to be born. Today Emily has ten nieces and nephews, twenty-five grandnieces and -nephews, and five great-grandnieces and -nephews, and knows each of them—where they are, what they're doing, how they differ, what traits they share.

Miss Eastman has had—and still has—many male friends, but she never quite married. "I've had attention from men," she reflects, "and I've had people in love with me. I've been more or less in love with some of them, as a matter of fact. But I've had rather bad luck. I mean the people I would really have liked to marry were either married themselves, or, well . . .

"There was one man in 1939, when I was visiting friends in South Africa. Actually I had known him when I was a child in England—he was 21 then, at Cambridge, and very nice to me; I thought him wonderful. He went back to South Africa and married. He had this business in Basutoland, which was then a protectorate, and really a delightful place. He had had a couple of children and his wife had died. He hadn't been too happy in the marriage.

"I went to visit, and the moment I looked at him I

thought he was still terribly attractive. By the end of the week he asked me to stay there and marry him. I was very much tempted; I was really quite nutty about him. But I said I'd got to go back to America and think this thing over at a distance.

"Well, I came back to New York, and of course the war broke out then. Also he was a shy person, himself convinced that anyone used to New York City or London couldn't possibly be happy in Ledingwana, Basutoland. But I'm quite sure I could have been."

Miss Eastman does not sound seriously regretful, however. "I do not believe, really, in fussing about how things *are,* or how they *might have been.* Of course sometimes I go over my life, and there are spots where I think, *If only I'd done such and such.* But I happen to be rather religious. And the older I get, the more I feel that God does ordain things, and that He probably knows what's what better than I do.

"My mother was a very wise person, I think, in her Victorian way. When I was a child and would complain that I didn't *want* to do something, or that I *wanted* something I couldn't have, she used to say, 'My dear, I can't see that *wanting* has anything to do with the matter!' "

In short, Miss Eastman has a way of accepting what comes and then getting on with the business of living, without fanfare or dramatics. This was true at the time of her first mastectomy. That she had cancer surprised her— "There'd never been *lumps* in my family, no one had ever had one!"—but she entered the hospital in calm spirits, informing neither relatives nor friends. "I knew perfectly well that if people knew, they would send cards and flowers—Americans do express themselves so frightfully in *things.* And I'd be visited in the hospital. There's nothing more tiring, I think. You have to be the hostess, or whatever you are; they're *there.*" The doctor nephew in Atlanta found out the truth, however, and phoned to say he was coming up to be with her. Touched but unpersuaded, Miss Eastman did her best to deter him. "*Countless* women have mastectomies, I told him; I told him it was a *very* common form of surgery." The nephew came anyway.

Despite all her traveling, Miss Eastman over the years has maintained her connection with the old ladies' home; only last year she was decorated by the Episcopal bishop for her many services. Recently the home vacated its quarters in Manhattan for a new building in the Bronx—"on the grounds of an old estate, a beautiful place, truly. But the old ladies don't like it—I still call them the old ladies, though most of them are younger than I am now.

"And no one wants to visit them now, because no one likes the subway ride. Oh, *I* go. And people say to me, 'You don't mean you go all the way up there by *subway!*' Well, I'm not enamored of the subway either, but I certainly can't afford to go by cab, so what's the matter with the subway then?"

Miss Eastman believes that many Americans are too concerned with being comfortable, that they would be better off in the long run if they couldn't always turn up the furnace or turn down the air conditioner, but endured a little more. In particular, she thinks Americans are overmedicated. She herself almost never takes a pill, except for a single aspirin when she feels a cold coming on. "That usually does the job."

She eats a light breakfast and lunch. She walks places. She sleeps beautifully and always has, even in London during the bombings. Every night at six she drinks a small glass of sherry and smokes a cigarette while watching the news. Her hand is steady, her mind calm and clear.

"I'm so well, I'm dull," says Emily Eastman cheerfully.

* * *

Though health profiling was never intended for people in their eighties, Miss Eastman wondered if there were not some way her risks could be assessed, and Dr. Charles M. Ross, of Interhealth, the San Diego profiling center, agreed to try an experiment. He suggested that she go ahead and submit her data. He would then process her through the computer as a 74-year-old, 74 being the upper age limit in the tables. Thus the results are not 100 percent valid—eleven extra years of age themselves constitute a risk. Nevertheless, Miss Eastman scored impressively. With her weight at 142 ("just about ideal," Dr. Ross says, for her 5'8" frame), and a blood pressure of only 140/80, her overall risks are those of a person of only 66, and are particularly low in the cardiovascular department, as can be seen below.

Note the cautionary observation concerning preexisting disease, in Emily's case breast cancer, for which no numerical risk factor can be assigned; Dr. Ross in his accompanying letter advises her, "Having had one cancer increases the risk for others and an annual sigmoidoscopic examination of the lower bowel would be helpful."

Note also that Miss Eastman lists herself as an ex-smoker. This is because years ago she used to smoke five or six cigarettes a day but is now down to one—the equivalent of not smoking, in her opinion. Ross is not completely convinced, but lets it pass: "This is an exciting Health Risk Profile; I wish I could see many more like it."

Here is Miss Eastman's profile:

HEALTH RISK PROFILE

Emily Eastman, age 85, white; processed as 74 years old.

Age in terms of present health, 66.

Achievable health age, 64.

OUTRANGING THE AGE TABLES

An average white woman of 74 has 34,153 chances per 100,000 of dying in the next ten years; your risks are 32% less than the average. You can, however, reduce these risks by 14%.

FACTORS OFFERING THE GREATEST REDUCTION IN RISK:	THE NUMBER OF YEARS TO BE GAINED BY ALTERING THOSE FACTORS:
Blood pressure	.8 year
Exercise	.5 year
Other factors	.7 year
Total	2.0 years

Your risks of death within the next ten years in descending importance:

1. ARTERIOSCLEROTIC HEART DISEASE (heart attack)

AVERAGE RISK	13,666 ●●●●●●●●●●
YOUR CURRENT RISK	5,330 ●●●●
YOUR ACHIEVABLE RISK	3,553 ●●●

INDICATORS OF RISK	RISK RATING	WAYS TO REDUCE RISK	RISK RATING
Current blood pressure 140/80	.6	Blood pressure 120/80 or less	.5
Current cholesterol not given—average used	1.0		
Diabetes—none	1.0		
Exercise—moderate	1.0	Exercise as directed	.8
Family history—none of early heart deaths	.9		
Former smoker	.9		
Weight 142 lbs.	.8		
History of abnormal electrocardiogram—none	1.0		
Current triglycerides not given—average used	1.0		

Excessive stress may increase risk. Exact risk factor not yet available.

2. STROKE

AVERAGE RISK	5,079 ●●●●●●●●●●
YOUR CURRENT RISK	3,047 ●●●●●●
YOUR ACHIEVABLE RISK	2,540 ●●●●●

INDICATORS OF RISK	RISK RATING	WAYS TO REDUCE RISK	RISK RATING
Current blood pressure 140/80	.6	Blood pressure 120/80	.5
Current cholesterol not given—average used	1.0		
Diabetes—none	1.0		
Former smoker	1.0		
History of abnormal electrocardiogram—none	1.0		

3. CANCER OF THE LARGE INTESTINE AND RECTUM

AVERAGE RISK	1,232 ●●●●●●●●●●
YOUR CURRENT RISK	1,232 ●●●●●●●●●●
YOUR ACHIEVABLE RISK	370 ●●●

INDICATORS OF RISK	RISK RATING	WAYS TO REDUCE RISK	RISK RATING
Intestinal polyps—none	1.0		
Rectal bleeding—none	1.0		
Ulcerative colitis—none	1.0		
Annual sigmoidoscopy—none	1.0	Annual in future	.3

4. BREAST CANCER (This patient has a history of the disease)

AVERAGE RISK	1,018 ●●●●●●●●●●
YOUR CURRENT RISK	1,018 ●●●●●●●●●●
YOUR ACHIEVABLE RISK	1,018 ●●●●●●●●●●

OUTRANGING THE AGE TABLES

Average risk is assigned because true risk factor is not known in cases where disease has occurred.

5. PNEUMONIA

AVERAGE RISK	777 ●●●●●●●●●●
YOUR CURRENT RISK	777 ●●●●●●●●●●
YOUR ACHIEVABLE RISK	777 ●●●●●●●●●●

INDICATORS OF RISK	RISK RATING	WAYS TO REDUCE RISK	RISK RATING
Alcohol consumption—3 to 6 drinks per week	1.0		
No history of bacterial pneumonia	1.0		
No history of emphysema	1.0		
Former smoker	1.0		

6. DISEASES OF THE ARTERIES

AVERAGE RISK	853 ●●●●●●●●●●
YOUR CURRENT RISK	512 ●●●●●●
YOUR ACHIEVABLE RISK	427 ●●●●●

INDICATORS OF RISK	RISK RATING	WAYS TO REDUCE RISK	RISK RATING
Current blood pressure 140/80	.6	Blood pressure 120/80 or less	.5
Current cholesterol not given—average used	1.0		
Diabetes—none	1.0		
Former smoker	1.0		

7. LUNG CANCER

AVERAGE RISK	564 ●●●●●●●●●●
YOUR CURRENT RISK	508 ●●●●●●●●●
YOUR ACHIEVABLE RISK	508 ●●●●●●●●●

THE LONGEVITY FACTOR

INDICATORS OF RISK	RISK RATING	WAYS TO REDUCE RISK	RISK RATING
Former smoker	.9		

8. CANCER OF THE OVARY

AVERAGE RISK	347 ●●●●●●●●●●
YOUR CURRENT RISK	347 ●●●●●●●●●●
YOUR ACHIEVABLE RISK	347 ●●●●●●●●●●

No risk indicators have been established for this cause of death.

9. BRONCHITIS AND EMPHYSEMA

AVERAGE RISK	314 ●●●●●●●●●●
YOUR CURRENT RISK	251 ●●●●●●●●
YOUR ACHIEVABLE RISK	251 ●●●●●●●●

INDICATORS OF RISK	RISK RATING	WAYS TO REDUCE RISK	RISK RATING
Former smoker	.8		
Lung function test not taken—average assumed	1.0		

10. HYPERTENSIVE HEART DISEASE

AVERAGE RISK	394 ●●●●●●●●●●
YOUR CURRENT RISK	189 ●●●●●
YOUR ACHIEVABLE RISK	158 ●●●●

INDICATORS OF RISK	RISK RATING	WAYS TO REDUCE RISK	RISK RATING
Current blood pressure 140/80	.6	Blood pressure 120/80 or less	.5
Weight 142 lbs.	.8		

OTHER

Your risk of death from all other causes in the next ten years totals 9,909 out of 100,000.

13

THE VERY BEST OF HEALTH: Jim Garro, Disturbing Family History

Every book, it is said, needs a hero. Ours has several— Ed Solomon, Kathleen Mooney, Dr. Eugene Howell, to name a few of the many who have worked to improve their health.

Then there is Jim Garro.

A management consultant by profession, partner in a large national firm, James F. Garro is six and a half feet in height, with longish sandy hair, tanned skin, very white whites in his eyes, and white, white teeth. At 33 he runs his firm's branch office in La Jolla, California, a place where he can enjoy the outdoors all year round and never has to wear a tie to the office, just an open-necked shirt, slacks, and sandals. Jim and his wife Claudia picked this location and this life after trying several cities in both the East and the Midwest. Jim says, "We finally decided we were going to live where we wanted to; if worst came to worst, I figured I could sell as many pencils as the next guy, maybe more."

He is a man who acts on his decisions. At the time he and Claudia became engaged, in 1968, in Connecticut, their home state, he told her, "When we get married, I'm going to get back into shape." At that point he weighed 225, 30 pounds more than he had when he played basketball in college.

He shed the extra avoirdupois by changing his diet, then, his interest aroused, began making a study of nutrition. Before long he gave up all sweets, all high-fat, high-cholesterol foods such as beef, pork, and eggs, and all so-called junk foods. When he travels by air these days, he even packs along his own lunch; the standard airline meals are, he says, "like putting paper in your mouth."

At the time of his marriage Jim also went back to exercising regularly, primarily running. This began as a kind of duty, then evolved into a pleasure, then into a necessity. Mornings in La Jolla now, he rises early, moving quietly so as not to wake his three small daughters, and runs five or six miles on the beach. He doesn't miss many mornings. "If I do, my body starts asking why, saying, 'Hey, I want you to take me out there and *run*.' " Traveling in Germany on business several years ago, he was hit by an automobile on a Berlin street, aggravating an old basketball knee injury so that he could not run, and he remembers the ensuing four months as the unhappiest period of his life, with doctors telling him he would have to get used to a sedentary existence. Instead, he sought out a famous sports surgeon and underwent a successful knee operation.

Happy, healthy, prosperous, still young, Jim nevertheless carries inside his brain an intimation of mortality. "I know I have genes floating around in my body that say 'High blood pressure.' My mom had it; so did her mom; so did her mom's mom—there's a long family history of strokes." But Garro himself doesn't intend to fall victim to a stroke or to any other form of cardiovascular disease—not if he can help it, and he believes that he can. Strokes and heart attacks, he says, "are the product of certain customs and mores in this country, which I don't have to share. I know what foods to eat now. I know how to exercise."

Two years ago he took up Transcendental Meditation because it was reputedly useful in lowering blood pressure, though his own blood pressure at the time was only 122/64. "I thought if I could get it down to 100 over 60, I would really like that." He also hopes to reduce his resting pulse rate to about 40—it's in the mid-50s now. Garro, incidentally, is also a practiced speed-reader.

Every year about the time of his birthday, Jim gets a health profile. He is now 33. This year his predicted risks were those of an 18-year-old—the best record yet for a person his age at the center which processed his profile.

HEALTH RISK PROFILE

Jim Garro, age 33, white.

Age in terms of present health, 18.

Achievable health age, 18.

An average white man your age has 2,170 chances per 100,000 of dying in the next ten years; your risks are 27% less than the average. You can reduce these risks by only .4%.

**Your risks of death within the next
ten years in descending importance:**

1. MOTOR VEHICLE ACCIDENTS

AVERAGE RISK	370	●●●●●●●●●●
YOUR CURRENT RISK	222	●●●●●●
YOUR ACHIEVABLE RISK	222	●●●●●●

THE VERY BEST OF HEALTH

INDICATORS OF RISK	RISK RATING	WAYS TO REDUCE RISK	RISK RATING
Alcohol consumption—3 to 6 drinks per week	.5		
Mileage yearly as driver or passenger—20,000	1.2		
Seat belt use—75% to 100% of time	.8		

2. SUICIDE

AVERAGE RISK	195 ●●●●●●●●●●
YOUR CURRENT RISK	195 ●●●●●●●●●●
YOUR ACHIEVABLE RISK	195 ●●●●●●●●●●

INDICATORS OF RISK	RISK RATING	WAYS TO REDUCE RISK	RISK RATING
Depression—no	1.0		
Family history of suicide—none	1.0		
Alcohol consumption—3 to 6 drinks per week	1.0		

3. HOMICIDE

AVERAGE RISK	130 ●●●●●●●●●●
YOUR CURRENT RISK	130 ●●●●●●●●●●
YOUR ACHIEVABLE RISK	130 ●●●●●●●●●●

INDICATORS OF RISK	RISK RATING	WAYS TO REDUCE RISK	RISK RATING
No arrests for violence	1.0		
Does not carry weapon	1.0		
Alcohol consumption—3 to 6 drinks per week	1.0		

THE LONGEVITY FACTOR

4. ACCIDENTS INVOLVING MACHINES (excluding cars)

AVERAGE RISK	67 ••••••••••
YOUR CURRENT RISK	67 ••••••••••
YOUR ACHIEVABLE RISK	67 ••••••••••

No risk indicators have been established for this cause of death.

5. AIRCRAFT ACCIDENTS

AVERAGE RISK	34 ••••••••••
YOUR CURRENT RISK	34 ••••••••••
YOUR ACHIEVABLE RISK	34 ••••••••••

No risk indicators have been established for this cause of death.

6. PNEUMONIA

AVERAGE RISK	34 ••••••••••
YOUR CURRENT RISK	34 ••••••••••
YOUR ACHIEVABLE RISK	34 ••••••••••

INDICATORS OF RISK	RISK RATING	WAYS TO REDUCE RISK	RISK RATING
Alcohol consumption—3 to 6 drinks per week	1.0		
No history of bacterial pneumonia	1.0		
No history of emphysema	1.0		
Nonsmoker	1.0		

7. FALLS

AVERAGE RISK	30 ●●●●●●●●●●
YOUR CURRENT RISK	30 ●●●●●●●●●●
YOUR ACHIEVABLE RISK	30 ●●●●●●●●●●

No risk indicators have been established for this cause of death.

8. BRAIN CANCER OR CANCER OF CENTRAL NERVOUS SYSTEM

AVERAGE RISK	28 ●●●●●●●●●●
YOUR CURRENT RISK	28 ●●●●●●●●●●
YOUR ACHIEVABLE RISK	28 ●●●●●●●●●●

No risk indicators have been established for this cause of death.

9. ARTERIOSCLEROTIC HEART DISEASE (heart attack)

AVERAGE RISK	292 ●●●●●●●●●●
YOUR CURRENT RISK	18 ●
YOUR ACHIEVABLE RISK	15 ●

INDICATORS OF RISK	RISK RATING	WAYS TO REDUCE RISK	RISK RATING
Current blood pressure 122/64	.5	Systolic blood pressure 120 or less	.4
Average of current and previous cholesterol 198	.7		
Diabetes—none	1.0		
Exercise—vigorous	.5		
Family history of early heart deaths—none	.9		
Nonsmoker	.5		
Weight—3% overweight	.8		
History of abnormal electrocardiogram— none	1.0		
Current triglycerides 70	1.0		

10. STROKE

AVERAGE RISK	62 ●●●●●●●●●●		
YOUR CURRENT RISK	15 ●●		
YOUR ACHIEVABLE RISK	12 ●●		

INDICATORS OF RISK	RISK RATING	WAYS TO REDUCE RISK	RISK RATING
Current blood pressure 122/64	.5	Systolic blood pressure 120 or less	.4
Current cholesterol 187	.6		
Diabetes—none	1.0		
Nonsmoker	.8		
History of abnormal electrocardiogram—none	1.0		

OTHER

Your risk of death from all other causes in the next ten years totals 805 out of 100,000.

PART III

14
CHANGING HABITS

With the possible exception of Emily Eastman, the assorted Americans you've just been reading about all undertook a common venture: the alteration of a deeply rooted habit, in some cases going back several decades. Almost all found the change difficult, and so, probably, will you (if indeed you haven't already, the last time you tried).

Habits, in truth, are profoundly personal things. In changing a habit, you're bidding goodbye to a part of yourself that you've long depended on, an old friend who celebrates triumphs with you, and consoles you for your defeats. Without your habit you are alone, unprotected.

Ridiculous? Maybe. Yet this is the way most habit changers feel in their first weeks. Depression and insomnia are common, sudden rages, ominous forebodings—even attacks of hypochondria, completely irrational when you consider that your new way of life can only make you healthier. But this very emphasis on health can itself be disturbing. For years you ate, drank, and smoked too much, confident that someone or something was taking care of you. Now you're taking care of yourself. You're vulnerable.

If changing a habit causes pain, moreover, it's pain that must be lived with and experienced, not just endured passively. To change, you must pay attention to what you're going through or you'll miss the positive signs, the moments of hope that do come, proving to you that you are not dying, but in fact moving forward. The new dieter, his meager lunch over, sets off down the sidewalk in a mood of depression—but discovers after several blocks that he is actually feeling sort of lively, in a strange way that has to do with the lean sensation in his midsection. Later, at dinner, the bleakness may return; yet that brisk walk happened, and lies there in his memory waiting for him to think of it; and on future days he can repeat it, noticing again how the exertion of walking along without too much food in the stomach is somehow invigorating; until the experience is no longer alien but becomes familiar, reassuring, and natural. The behavioral vacuum is beginning to fill in. Here is a part of the new self that he is slowly becoming.

* * *

If you want to change a habit, try breaking the process into three stages. The first is investigative.

Exploring the Change

What you're engaged in, in effect, is a study of how to live in order to function well physically. Don't cut the study short. Let it run on a month, if necessary—however long it takes to come to a clear understanding of the handicap under which your body is laboring.

Jack Kodaly, if you will remember, actually followed a similar process, but with a very different attitude which may have increased his suffering. Month after month Jack resolved each day not to smoke, then castigated himself bitterly when he yielded to temptation. Yet he was making a growing breach in his habit, smoking a little less all the time. Perhaps if he had labeled his efforts "exploratory" he would have felt more sense of progress, even gained his freedom a little sooner.

Say that you, like Jack, want to stop smoking. Start out not by renouncing all cigarettes, but by finding out what nonsmoking feels like in different situations. First, try omitting the cigarette you used to smoke at bedtime, then the one you've always had with coffee. One day you'll go all morning without smoking and survive; another day you'll smoke in the morning but refrain in the evening.

This process is sometimes called tapering off, but there is much more to it than simply decreasing your quota of cigarettes. You are learning what you are getting yourself into, before making a permanent commitment. And you are starting small, where success comes easy.

During this preparatory period you should also begin developing substitutes for your habit, using them deliberately and consistently so that when quitting time comes they will be well established in your life and ready to help you. Giving up butter on bread (to lose weight, or to lower cholesterol and/or triglycerides) may be virtually impossible, but replacing the butter with low-fat cottage cheese is not. Respiratory activities like running or singing do help fill the physical vacuum of not smoking—running in particular. You may at first deride it as a combination of masochism and narcissism, but running has helped millions of people to change their lives.

This matter of the substitute or replacement habit is crucial to successful changing, though it is sometimes passed over lightly. Why, really, do people smoke, drink, and overeat? Because these are means for rewarding themselves. Often they don't realize this until they try to stop—only to discover that their daily life has mysteriously lost its incentives.

A person can learn to live without sweets, without cigarettes, without alcohol, but no one can live without a reward system. What you must do is build a new one. For most people, this means putting together a bundle of different rewards, to be taken out and used as circumstance requires.

First, you'll need in some fashion to replace those purely tactile rewards that you're used to experiencing when you indulge your habit. For drinkers, smokers, and overeaters alike, these have to do mainly with the lips, mouth, and throat and are usually summed up in the term oral gratification. It is for oral gratification that the habit changer chomps away on radishes, sucks lemons, pours glass after glass of ice water down his quailing throat, and chews gum until his jaws ache. Some find peace in brushing their teeth. Others sing, or even cry. Pick out three or four such substitutes that you think might be of help to you and start cultivating them. In making your selection, however, remember you may be paving the way for a brand new addiction of one sort or another, so be cautious. Jack Kodaly, if he chose, could eat a pound of sunflower seeds a day without doing himself harm; Kathleen Mooney, on the other hand, suddenly found herself gulping down dangerous amounts of Darvon, a powerful prescription drug.

Second, you'll want to devise new ways to relax. This is truest for people who stop drinking, alcohol being a pharmacological depressant. But nicotine, though technically a stimulant, also soothes, smokers insist; and perhaps any habit, just because it rewards you, is automatically relaxing.

During this first exploratory stage, therefore, take ten minutes or so several times a day to practice the art of relaxing. Essentially this means letting the muscles flop, breathing slowly, and thinking soothing thoughts. This is easy enough to achieve if you're feeling at peace with the

CHANGING HABITS

world anyway and have a comfortable bed to stretch out on; what you need is to develop the technique to the point where it can help you through a crisis. Practice relaxing while sitting up in a chair, while standing, and under various adverse conditions, such as a traffic jam or following a quarrel with a friend. If you run into difficulties consult one of the many self-help books on the subject (a good one is *The Relaxation Response* by Dr. Herbert Benson) and/or join a Yoga class.

Meditation twice a day helps many people stay generally relaxed, while others like a warm bath (just lie in it for half an hour, letting your thoughts drift). As for pills—tranquilizers—these, too, can lower tension but have not proved particularly helpful in changing habits, perhaps because they encourage a mood of dependency in the user at a time when self-control and self-management are what is needed. In addition, tranquilizers can become a habit themselves, and a hard one to break.

The exploratory stage in habit changing is also the time to take inventory of your personal interests, selecting those strong enough to help pull you through your first weeks. What you want is an activity you can turn to that is capable of suddenly and totally changing the subject inside your head, whether that subject be a chocolate ice cream cone, a bottle of vodka, or a Marlboro 100. Did you ever stay up past midnight to finish a crossword puzzle? Start weeding the garden—and go on even when it rained? Sit down to play the piano for a few minutes, and suddenly realize an hour had passed? Tennis, needlework, even cleaning closets, as Don Hanson's friend discovered: these are all activities that people tend to become addictive about—and that are, therefore, strong enough to blot out temptation.

Jigsaw puzzles? Why not? The day before you quit, go buy yourself the biggest, hardest jigsaw puzzle you can find. Empty it out on a card table. It will be there waiting to obsess you, in those moments when an obsession is the only thing that eases your pain.

Then save it for those moments. This is important, not only with jigsaw puzzles, but with all your new-found remedies. If you nibble celery and carrots all day long, you'll get so sick of them they won't help any more; save them, instead, for a certain time of day—maybe midmorning. In your office, don't keep getting up to pace restlessly; instead, take one long walk at lunch hour. Don't haunt the water cooler; do have tea or tomato juice at four o'clock. Don't keep muttering *Relax!* to yourself, but two or three times a day do relax, as completely as you know how, for ten full minutes. Station the islands of interest, islands of refuge, throughout your day, so you'll always have something to look ahead to. This is how old habits are dropped—by forging new ones.

And by forging new attitudes. Dr. Ralph Hylinski of California State University in Hayward, California, has worked with many students who tried to give up smoking. He says, "I ask them to think about one little word: *forever*. Can they say to themselves, 'I want to stop smoking *forever*'? Those that can are ready. The rest—well, they may try just as hard, but their success rate is much lower."

Then there is Dr. Herbert Spiegel. Dr. Spiegel is a New York psychiatrist who teaches at Columbia University's College of Physicians and Surgeons, and who uses hypnosis to help people with smoking and weight problems.

The first thing smokers must realize, Spiegel says, is that their identity doesn't begin and end with smoking. Smoking is only one of many attributes belonging to a person; what he or she can learn to do is to use the other attributes, such as executive skills, to *stop* smoking. But it can't be done by fighting cigarettes. "That's like deciding not to swallow," says Spiegel. "You know, the harder you try, the more you need to swallow."

CHANGING HABITS

Dr. Spiegel uses hypnosis not to issue commands, but to alter attitudes, to get his patients' minds off the subject of cigarettes and onto the subject of their bodily well-being. He helps a patient to enter a light trance. Then, very slowly and clearly, he begins to speak:

"Point number one: for your body, smoking is a poison. You are composed of a number of components, the most important of which is your body. Smoking is not so much a poison for *you*, as it is for your body specifically.

"The second point: You cannot live without your body. Your body is a precious physical plant through which *you* experience life.

"The third point: To the extent that you want to live, you owe your body respect and protection.

"You are in truth your body's keeper.

"When you make this commitment to respect your body, you have within you the power to have smoked your last cigarette."

Some patients, Spiegel says, are chagrined to discover that hypnosis is no magic charm in habit change. "They come in thinking that in some way I'm going to make them quit, without any effort on their part. Then after a while, the light dawns. They say, 'Hey wait a minute, you expect *me* to do this thing?' "

In fact Spiegel, who calls the whole process restructuring, puts strong emphasis on a spirit of initiative and personal responsibility; he says it's the only spirit that works. He keeps his office well supplied with ashtrays, for instance, on the premise that it's the patient's decision, not his, whether to smoke or not. Moreover, he usually deals with smokers in just one 45-minute treatment. "When they come in that first time, if I were to indicate, 'Well, we'll try this out, and if it doesn't work, then we'll try some other way,' there would never be a moment of confrontation. And the next thing you know, they'd be involved in this ceremony of going to a doctor, thinking that somehow, some way, they're going to change. That's nonsense.

"But if I take the approach, 'This is it, Buster—it's all in one session,' it's truly amazing how serious people can get." Instead of repeat treatments, Spiegel uses his single session to teach patients how to maintain their new attitudes through *self*-hypnosis, to be practiced in frequent, very brief snatches, both at work and at home, throughout the early weeks of change.*

Making the Change

After all the preparation, the first few days on a diet (or off alcohol or cigarettes) can be reassuring, in spite of the pain. You've entered your program at last. Now you're actually doing something. And pretty soon, you remind yourself, the rewards will start coming in: lost pounds, lowered cholesterol, cough-free mornings, whatever it is that you're looking forward to. Impatiently you await the first good signs, clinging firmly to your resolve, looking neither right nor left.

Of course you feel tense and nervous, but many of the worst symptoms these first few days are essentially physiological as your body, knowing no better, reacts with dismay to the change. If you've been drinking 20 ounces of 90-proof alcohol daily for a period of years, that is what your physical plant accepts as normal, even necessary; when you cut off the supply, alarms start ringing all over your body—shakiness, sweating, insomnia. The dieter suffers.hideous, yearning sensations in his midriff; the ex-smoker feels like he's drowning in air. But most people who have prepared properly can survive this kind of dis-

---

* Dr. Spiegel has published a book, written in collaboration with his son, also a physician, *Trance and Treatment—Clinical Uses of Hypnosis*, by Herbert Spiegel and David Spiegel, published by Basic Books, Inc., New York, 1978.

tress. They know where they're going, and their momentum is strong.

During these first days, it's important to:

1. Put into daily practice the new activities and techniques that you developed during your preparatory stage.
2. Stay active and busy, but with islands of rest and relaxation.
3. Avoid emotional buildups inside yourself. Try to talk often, using not only your voice and mouth but your emotions.
4. Keep physically active. Exercise is one of the surest outlets for tension.
5. Plan each day in advance, at a time when you're feeling calm, such as on first waking up in the morning. Write down what you're going to do, then spend your day accomplishing the items one by one. Circle any that you look forward to, even if it's only a bath. Daily planning helps restore the feeling of structure that your habit used to give you. It also tells you what to do in moments of panic.
6. When the suffering strikes, don't tense up and fight back. Accept it, more or less as you would accept the discomfort of a bad cold, reminding yourself that it will pass and that you are headed in the right direction.

Joining a group—as Kathleen Mooney and Don Hanson joined AA, Laura Blake Smokenders, and Ed Solomon the Pritikin Clinic in Santa Barbara—can be an immense help and often makes the difference between stopping for only a day or two, and staying stopped.[*] You need people to turn to who will be sympathetic but not pitying, who can understand your torment and simultaneously support your determination. Your fellow habit-changers will offer you advice about your specific difficulties, and you in turn can advise them about theirs—which also benefits you, because

---

[*] Lucille Meeker's only major progress in her repeated efforts to lose weight came during her enrollment in a group, Weight Watchers.

it gives you a kind of objectivity about the common problem. You're going through the same thing together, and together you can win.

Groups also teach you systematic methods to follow in changing a habit. And of course they give you meetings to go to—that is, opportunities to get away from your usual haunts, which all too often serve only to remind you of the substance you're struggling to live without. Alcoholics Anonymous, in particular, recognizes the need not only for advice and solace, but for someplace to go, something to do, to fill in the many hours that once were devoted to drinking. In metropolitan areas today, an ex-drinker can usually find an AA meeting to attend every night of the week, plus three or four on weekends. Weight Watchers also tries to make meetings available to its members virtually every night.

The first days of habit change are stormy, difficult, and, above all, full of uncertainty. Lapses, if they occur, are devastating. Real confidence builds slowly, and builds only on success. It comes, though, at last, one day, if you hang on long enough—that assurance, that calmness, that says, with something like a sigh, "I did it." In this moment you realize not only that you *can* change, but that you *are* changing; you *have* changed.

Naturally you're tremendously pleased with yourself. Aren't you? You look about you. You see a healthy future stretching out ahead. Then suddenly you ask yourself, "Was *this* what I wanted?" Welcome to stage 3 of habit changing.

Maintaining the Change

Your first thrust is spent now, the high drama over. You no longer burst into tears if you can't find the car keys, or feel like jumping out a window when the phone rings. You're living without your habit, and surviving. You even feel fairly calm about it all.

Then why aren't you more grateful?

Stage 3 is the most dangerous stage, a fact confirmed by many statistical studies of habit-change programs. Figures from these studies vary widely, but the general trend is unmistakable: a high initial success rate, followed by a steady and dismal dwindling away in the months that follow, until after a year or two very little is left to crow about. Typical is one study of the highly respected smoking-cessation clinics run by Seventh-Day Adventists: it was found that 75 to 80 percent of the participants stopped smoking, but only 34 percent stayed stopped as long as three months, and only 15 to 20 percent lasted a year.

The problems of stage 3 are almost exclusively mental, but they are extremely tricky to handle. Sure you feel better physically. But that dim sense of deprivation can persist and persist. Many people at this point begin to feel lonely, almost scared, as if they have somehow progressed farther and faster than they really meant to. Can't they turn back one last time, just to touch base?

It was in this state of mind that Lucille Meeker, after losing 25 pounds, went out and bought a dish of maple walnut ice cream. *Just this once,* she said to herself.

So we meekly reason our way backward, into the very habit from which we thought we'd freed ourselves.

Similar results can be achieved by moralizing. *I've been good for two whole months!* you suddenly say to yourself— by which you mean that to lower your cholesterol, you've eaten nothing but cottage cheese and raw vegetables (and precious little of those). In a burst of euphoria you add, *Why, I'm going to be good all year!* A helpful, positive approach to your problem? Not necessarily. For what happens when the year ends? As sure as the tides change, people eventually have got to be "bad" again. And if your way of being bad is to eat butter and eggs, there goes your cholesterol reduction program.

Others moralize more negatively. *Why am I suffering so?* they ask themselves. *Because I'm being punished for my weakness, that's why. And I deserve to be punished. For years I did nothing but indulge myself.*

But punishment, like virtue, can't last forever. Sooner or later your conscience takes pity on you. You've deprived yourself for so long. Now it's time to do something nice—like smoke a cigarette, "just one."

Changing a habit is a matter of making choices—not only the single choice at the beginning ("I will never drink again"), but choices over and over again, day after day. You choose each morning not to drink that day, and you must reinforce your decision all day long—at lunch, when you order iced tea instead of a martini, after work when a friend suggests you drop in at a bar, or back home watching television.

As the weeks pass the choice becomes easier, particularly when you fill in the vacuum of not drinking with other activities. For a long time, though, for some people, once in a while, the "wrong" choice will happen. This doesn't have to mean disaster. The idea that "once you lapse, you're lost" is one of those unfortunate misconceptions, true only if you let it be true. If you find yourself backsliding, keep calm and at least try to learn something. Pay attention to what you're experiencing. A candy bar, if you haven't consumed one in six months, may taste surprising, not necessarily so delicious as you remembered. Pizza, after a long absence, can feel heavy and oily in the stomach.

Or maybe the physical sensations will be pleasant, but even then there'll be a difference, a curious feeling of unfamiliarity, and that is what to concentrate on. You have moved a considerable distance out from under your habit;

it's no longer a part of you. Above all, recognize that your backslide didn't just happen but was a matter of choice, a choice *you* made, just as you can make the "right" choice next time, and the time after.

In maintaining your change, beware of overconfidence. Stay humble, and use any help you can get. Recognize that an appetite that you've been reinforcing daily for twenty years or more is not going to die out in a month or two. Instead it goes underground, biding its time till your defenses are down.

After the first few weeks, you may think that you no longer need the daily routines you worked on in your initial preparations—the relaxation drills, the oral substitutes, the special activities. Practice them anyway, at least a few times a week, oftener when you find yourself feeling edgy or deprived. The more you use them to reward yourself, the more rewarding they will become. And keep going to the group meetings if they help you. Remember, unless you can make your new life more satisfying than the old one, you aren't going to want to continue it, no matter how strong your willpower.

To change a powerful habit, you need a powerful motive. Gene Howell thought he could not survive a day without cigarettes, until he learned he had lung cancer; then his craving vanished as if it had never existed. Kathleen Mooney in her alcoholic misery, Ed Solomon living a life of pain and fear because of angina—these are people who had strong reasons to change.

What about your reasons? Will they stand up through hard times ahead? This is a subject to think about seriously —and a good place to start the thought process is at your desk, as you read carefully through your health profile.

PART IV

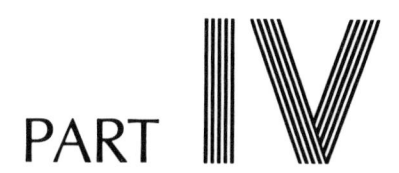

This section will guide you to your own personal health profile, with a choice of three alternative methods. In Chapter 15 you'll find a rudimentary quick quiz, a kind of basic introduction to the health profiling process. Chapter 16 reprints a standard health profile questionnaire exactly as it comes from the data center, the kind you can fill out and submit for computer processing. Chapter 17 tells you how to calculate your health profile by yourself.

15

YOUR OWN HEALTH PROFILE: The Short Form

In 1976 the Canadian government mailed out a copy of the questionnaire that follows to more than 3 million Canadians on social security, after a test run indicated that fully a third of the recipients could be expected to modify unhealthy habits, at least temporarily; subsequent observation has confirmed this prediction.

This quiz may do the same thing for you, perhaps even permanently:

HOW HEALTHY IS YOUR LIFE STYLE?

Circle only the answers that apply to you, either on the left, in the center, or on the right.

The plus and minus signs next to some numbers indicate more than (+) and less than (−).

Exercise

Physical effort expended during the workday: mostly
Heavy labor, Walking, Housework | Deskwork

Participation in physical activities—skiing, golf, swimming, etc., or lawn mowing, gardening, etc.?
Daily | Weekly | Seldom

Participation in a vigorous exercise program?
3 times weekly | Weekly | Seldom

Average miles walked or jogged per day?
1 or more | less than 1 | None

Flights of stairs climbed per day?
10 plus | fewer than 10 | ———

Nutrition

Are you overweight?
No | 5 to 19 lbs. | 20+ lbs.

Do you eat a wide variety of ...omething from each of the ...ng five food groups: (1) meat, fish, poultry, dried legumes, eggs or nut... ... milk products; (3) bread or cereals; (4) fruits; (5) vegetables?
Each day | 3 times weekly |

Alcohol

Average number of bottles (12 oz.) of beer per week?
0 to 7 | 8 to 15 | 16+

Average number hard liquor (1½ oz.) drinks per week?
0 to 7 | 8 to 15 | 16+

Average number of glasses (5 oz.) of wine or cider per week?
0 to 7 | 8 to 15 | 16+

Total number of drinks per week, including beer, liquor and wine?
0 to 7 | 8 to 15 | 16+

Drugs

Do you take drugs illegally?
No | | Yes

Do you consume alcoholic beverages together with certain drugs (tranquilizers, barbiturates, illegal drugs)?
No | | Yes

Do you use pain-killers improperly or excessively?
No | | Yes

Tobacco

Cigarettes smoked per day?
None | fewer than 10 | 10+

YOUR OWN HEALTH PROFILE: The Short Form

Cigars smoked per day?
None | fewer than 5 | 5+

Pipe tobacco pouches per week?
None | fewer than 2 | 2+

Personal Health

Do you experience periods of depression?
Seldom | Occasionally | Frequently

Does anxiety interfere with your daily activities?
No | Occasionally | Frequently

Do you get enough satisfying sleep?
Yes | No | —

Are you aware of the causes and dangers of VD?
Yes | No | —

Breast self-examination? (If not applicable, do not score.)
Monthly | Occasionally | —

Road and Water Safety

Mileage per year as driver or passenger?
10,000− | 10,000+ |

Do you often exceed the speed limit?
No | by 10 mph+ | by 20 mph+

Do you wear a seat belt?
Always | Occasionally | Never

Do you drive a motorcycle, moped or snowmobile?
No | Yes |

If yes to the above, do you always wear a regulation safety helmet?
Yes | | No

Do you ever drive under the influence of alcohol?
Never | | Occasionally

Do you ever drive when your ability may be affected by drugs?
Never | | Occasionally

Are you aware of water-safety rules?
Yes | No |

If you participate in water sports or boating, do you wear a life jacket?
Yes | No |

General

Average time watching TV per day (in hours)?
0 to 1 | 1 to 4 | 4+

Are you familiar with first-aid procedures?
Yes | No |

Do you ever smoke in bed?
No | Occasionally | Yes

Do you always make use of equipment provided for your safety at work?
Yes | Occasionally | No

TO SCORE: Give yourself 1 point for each answer in column 1; 3 points for each answer in column 2; 5 points for each answer in column 3.
TOTAL SCORE _____

How to Calculate Your Score
Excellent 34−45
You have a commendable lifestyle based on sensible habits and a lively awareness of personal health.

THE LONGEVITY FACTOR

HOW HEALTHY IS YOUR LIFE STYLE? (cont.)

Good: 46–55
With some minor change, you can develop an excellent lifestyle.

Risky: 56–65
You are taking unnecessary risks with your health. Several of your habits should be changed if potential health problems are to be avoided.

Hazardous: 66 and over
Either you have little personal awareness of good health habits, or you are choosing to ignore them. This is a danger zone.

16

YOUR OWN HEALTH PROFILE: Computer-Assisted

Obtaining the most complete and detailed health profile involves filling out the stock questionnaire of one of the several existing medical data centers offering this service. You send the questionnaire in by mail, and the resulting profile will come back to you in an envelope marked confidential. The "confidential" is serious: since these computer centers are run by medical doctors, their oath of practice permits them to divulge such personal information only to patients, unless the patients direct them to release it.

Here are the mailing addresses of five centers equipped to process their own questionnaires:

- General Health, P.O. Box 573-46, Washington, D.C. 20037
- Institute for Life Style Improvement, University of Wisconsin, Stevens Point, Wis. 54481
- Interhealth, 2970 Fifth Avenue, San Diego, Calif. 92103
- Medical Datamation, Southwest and Harrison Streets, Bellevue, Ohio 44811

- Methodist Hospital of Indiana, Prospective Health Department, Indianapolis, Ind. 46202
- Wellness Resources Center, 126 Hillside, Mill Valley, Calif. 94941

Each of these organizations provides a questionnaire kit upon request; in some cases, you can also arrange to send blood samples for chemical testing. Or, if that is difficult, you will be asked to find out your cholesterol level, blood pressure, triglyceride count, and other information from your private physician or company doctor and to enter the figures on the appropriate lines of the questionnaire. The alternative is to leave those questions unanswered, in which case an average figure will be assigned you, but the more precise information given, the truer the result.

A computerized health profile is not expensive: among the centers listed, the present range of costs starts at three dollars. You can still do it all yourself, however, with only a little less precision, by following the directions on page 223.

The questionnaire we've chosen to reproduce (turned sideways, it occupies the next fifteen pages) is from Interhealth of San Diego, which has processed the profiles used in the rest of this book; the questionnaire is printed by permission of the copyright owners, Control Data Corporation, of which Interhealth is a division.

YOUR OWN HEALTH PROFILE: Computer-Assisted

Your answers to the questions that follow will allow us to attempt to give *you* clues, to some of the greatest risks to your survival over the next 10-year period of your life. By compiling your present risks and estimating your future risks, we may be able to help *you* begin a series of procedures to reduce these risks.

Please answer every question. All questions, even those that inquire about race or religion, are asked *only* because they are associated with different risks in certain diseases.

INSTRUCTIONS FOR COMPLETING THESE QUESTIONS
PLEASE USE A PENCIL ONLY

- Mark a cross in the box ☒ opposite your answer.
- If you change an answer, *please erase the cross* completely before marking your corrected answer.
- Be sure to answer every question.

PATIENT IDENTIFICATION

Please print the first two letters of your last name here. 224 ☐☐

Birthdate: 219 ☐☐ ☐☐ ☐☐ Sex: 220 ☐ Male 221 ☐ Female
MONTH DAY YEAR

Weight (Pounds): 222 ☐☐☐ Height: 223 _____ Feet _____ Inches

203

OCCUPATION: _____
(such as Housewife, Secretary, Salesperson, Actor, Electrician, Farmer, Health Services, Miner, Lawyer, Carpenter, etc.)

PRESENT MARITAL STATUS

- 231 ☐ Single
- 232 ☐ Married
- 233 ☐ Divorced
- 234 ☐ Widowed
- 235 ☐ Separated
- 236 ☐ Remarried

Has there been a change in marital status in the past year?

- 237 ☐ No
- 238 ☐ Yes

DO YOU LIVE

- 239 ☐ Alone
- 240 ☐ With spouse, family or relatives
- 241 ☐ With friends
- 242 ☐ In nursing or boarding home in the last 6 months
- 243 ☐ Other

LENGTH OF TIME AT PRESENT JOB, OR, IF UNEMPLOYED, AT LAST JOB

- 244 ☐ 1 year or less
- 245 ☐ 1-5 years
- 246 ☐ Over 5 years

EDUCATION *(SCHOOLING)*
Mark the one box opposite the last year completed.

Grade School	247 ☐ 1	248 ☐ 2	249 ☐ 3	250 ☐ 4	251 ☐ 5	252 ☐ 6	253 ☐ 7	254 ☐ 8
High School	255 ☐ 1	256 ☐ 2	257 ☐ 3	258 ☐ 4				
Beyond High School	259 ☐ 1	260 ☐ 2	261 ☐ 3	262 ☐ 4	263 ☐ 5 or more			

YOUR OWN HEALTH PROFILE: Computer-Assisted

PLEASE MARK THE ONE ANSWER THAT BEST DESCRIBES HOW MUCH EXERCISE OR PHYSICAL ACTIVITY YOU GET INCLUDING YOUR WORK.

- 009 ☐ Climbing less than five flights of stairs or walking less than ½ mile four times per week, or other equal activity.
- 010 ☐ Climbing 5 - 5 flights of stairs or walking ½ - 1½ miles four times per week, or other equal activity.
- 011 ☐ Climbing 15-20 flights of stairs or walking 1½ - 2 miles four times per week, or other equal activity.
- 012 ☐ Exercise greater than any of these.

HAVE EITHER OF YOUR NATURAL PARENTS (MOTHER OR FATHER) DIED BEFORE AGE 60 OF HEART TROUBLE?

- 013 ☐ No   014 ☐ Yes   IF YES, MARK THE ONE CORRECT ANSWER:
  - 015 ☐ One parent died before age 60 of heart trouble.
  - 016 ☐ Both parents died before age 60 of heart trouble.

HAVE YOU EVER BEEN TOLD THAT YOU HAD DIABETES *(TOO MUCH SUGAR IN THE BLOOD)*?

- 017 ☐ No   018 ☐ Yes   IF YES, MARK ALL CORRECT ANSWERS:
  - 019 ☐ I follow a diet for diabetes.
  - 020 ☐ I take insulin (shots) for diabetes.
  - 021 ☐ I take pills for diabetes.
  - 022 ☐ None of these.

HAVE YOUR NATURAL PARENTS (MOTHER OR FATHER), BROTHERS OR SISTERS HAD DIABETES?

- 023 ☐ No   024 ☐ Yes

HAVE YOU EVER HAD CHEST X-RAYS?

- 025 ☐ No   026 ☐ Yes   IF YES, MARK ALL CORRECT ANSWERS ABOUT THE X-RAYS:
  - 027 ☐ They were not normal.
  - 028 ☐ I don't know the result.
  - 029 ☐ Some were normal, some were not normal.
  - 030 ☐ The X-ray was normal within the past 12 months.
  - 225 ☐ None of these.

205

MARK YOUR RACE

215 ☐ Black   216 ☐ Red   217 ☐ White   218 ☐ Yellow   228 ☐ Other _____

DO YOU HAVE SICKLE CELL ANEMIA?

229 ☐ No   230 ☐ Yes

HAVE YOU EVER HAD AN ECG *(EKG, ELECTROCARDIOGRAM, HEART TRACING)*?

031 ☐ No   032 ☐ Yes   IF YES, MARK ALL CORRECT ANSWERS:

033 ☐ It was not normal within 3 years.
034 ☐ Some were normal, some were not normal.
035 ☐ They were all normal.
036 ☐ I don't know the result.
037 ☐ None of these.

HAVE YOU EVER BEEN TOLD YOU HAD TROUBLE WITH YOUR HEART?

264 ☐ No   265 ☐ Yes   IF YES, MARK ALL ANSWERS THAT SEEM LIKE WHAT WAS SAID ABOUT YOUR HEART:

266 ☐ It was a heart murmur or a leaky heart.
267 ☐ It was rheumatic fever.
268 ☐ It was angina or angina pectoris.
269 ☐ It was a heart attack or coronary.

DO YOU TAKE PENICILLIN OR MEDICINE LIKE IT TO PREVENT HEART INFECTION OR RHEUMATIC FEVER?

007 ☐ No   008 ☐ Yes

HAVE YOU EVER BEEN TOLD YOU HAD HIGH BLOOD PRESSURE?

270 ☐ No   271 ☐ Yes   IF YES, WHAT WAS YOUR HIGHEST BLOOD PRESSURE? 272 _____

HAVE YOU TAKEN ANY MEDICINE FOR YOUR HEART OR BLOOD PRESSURE DURING THE PAST 6 MONTHS?

273 ☐ No   274 ☐ Yes

YOUR OWN HEALTH PROFILE: Computer-Assisted

DO YOU NOW SMOKE?

038 ☐ No   039 ☐ Yes

IF YES, MARK ALL CORRECT ANSWERS:

I smoke:

- 040 ☐ Cigarettes - 2 or more packs per day.
- 041 ☐ Cigarettes - 1½ packs per day.
- 042 ☐ Cigarettes - 1 pack per day.
- 043 ☐ Cigarettes - ½ pack per day.
- 044 ☐ Cigarettes - less than ½ pack per day.
- 045 ☐ Cigars or pipe - 5 or more per day (combined total).
- 046 ☐ Cigars or pipe - less than 5 per day (combined total).

DID YOU SMOKE, BUT NO LONGER DO?

047 ☐ No   048 ☐ Yes

IF YES,

How long ago did you stop? 049 _____ years ago

If less than one year — 050 _____ months ago

IF YOU DID SMOKE, MARK ALL CORRECT ANSWERS:

I smoked:

- 051 ☐ Cigarettes - 2 or more packs per day.
- 052 ☐ Cigarettes - 1½ packs per day.
- 053 ☐ Cigarettes - 1 pack per day.
- 054 ☐ Cigarettes - ½ pack per day.
- 055 ☐ Cigarettes - less than ½ pack per day.
- 056 ☐ Cigars or pipe - 5 or more per day (combined total).
- 057 ☐ Cigars or pipe - less than 5 per day (combined total).

HAVE YOU EVER BEEN TOLD YOU HAD LUNG TROUBLE OR BREATHING TROUBLE?

058 ☐ No   059 ☐ Yes   IF YES, MARK ALL CORRECT ANSWERS:

060 ☐ The trouble was emphysema.
061 ☐ The trouble was pneumonia.
062 ☐ I had tuberculosis (TB, consumption).
063 ☐ I am being treated for tuberculosis now.
064 ☐ None of these.

HAVE YOU HAD A SKIN TEST FOR TB (TUBERCULOSIS, CONSUMPTION) IN THE PAST YEAR?

065 ☐ No   066 ☐ Yes   IF YES, MARK ALL CORRECT ANSWERS:

067 ☐ It was negative or normal.
068 ☐ It became positive or not normal this year.
069 ☐ It was positive this year and also before that.
070 ☐ None of these.

IN THE PAST SIX (6) MONTHS HAVE YOU HAD BLEEDING FROM YOUR RECTUM *(WHERE YOUR BOWEL MOVEMENTS COME OUT)*?

071 ☐ No   072 ☐ Yes

HAVE YOU HAD A FINGER EXAMINATION OF YOUR RECTUM *(WHERE YOUR BOWEL MOVEMENTS COME OUT)* BY YOUR DOCTOR IN THE PAST YEAR?

073 ☐ No   074 ☐ Yes

HAVE YOU HAD AN EXAMINATION OF YOUR RECTUM OR COLON BY YOUR DOCTOR WITH A LIGHTED INSTRUMENT IN THE PAST YEAR (SIGMOIDOSCOPY, PROCTO, PROCTOSCOPY)?

075 ☐ No   076 ☐ Yes

HAVE YOU EVER HAD POLYPS (SMALL TUMORS) OR GROWTHS IN YOUR INTESTINE OR RECTUM (NOT PILES OR HEMORRHOIDS)?

077 ☐ No   078 ☐ Yes

YOUR OWN HEALTH PROFILE: Computer-Assisted

DO YOU HAVE ULCERATIVE COLITIS *(BLOODY DIARRHEA WITH PUS AND MUCOUS AND SORES INSIDE THE RECTUM)?*

079 ☐ No   **080** ☐ Yes   IF YES, MARK HOW LONG YOU HAVE HAD IT:

081 ☐ More than 10 years
082 ☐ 10 years or less

HOW MANY TOTAL MILES PER YEAR DO YOU TRAVEL IN A CAR OR MOTOR VEHICLE AS A DRIVER OR PASSENGER?

083 _____ miles per year.

To help you in estimating the number of miles you drive or ride, the national averages for the following categories of driving are listed below:

Driving to and from work — 8000 miles per year.
Driving to and from shopping and other personal business — 4000 miles per year.
Driving to and from school and church — 1000 miles per year.
Driving to and from pleasure, recreation and miscellaneous — 5000 miles per year.

HOW MANY OF THESE MILES ARE ON A FREEWAY, EXPRESSWAY, TOLL ROAD OR OTHER SIMILAR LIMITED ACCESS HIGHWAY?

084 ☐ Most (75% or more)   **085** ☐ Some (25-74%)   **086** ☐ Little (0-24%)

WHEN IN A MOTOR VEHICLE (CAR), DO YOU WEAR A SEAT BELT OR SHOULDER HARNESS?

087 ☐ No   **088** ☐ Yes   IF YES, MARK WHEN YOU WEAR IT:

089 ☐ Less than 10% of the time.
090 ☐ 10 - 24% of the time.
091 ☐ 25 - 74% of the time.
092 ☐ 75% or more of the time.

209

MARK ANY OF THESE THAT YOU DO:

- 093 ☐ Fly a private plane
- 094 ☐ Sky dive
- 095 ☐ Skin dive - scuba dive
- 096 ☐ Drive a racing car, dune buggy, snowmobile, or motorcycle in dirt (off the road)
- 227 ☐ Drive a motorcycle on the street

MARK ANY OF THE MEDICINES YOU ARE NOW TAKING

- 097 ☐ Mood elevators (pills of depression)
- 098 ☐ Pep or diet pills (like dexadrine)
- 099 ☐ Tranquilizers, sedatives, nerve or sleeping pills (Miltown, Librium, Phenobarbital, Nembutal, Seconal, etc.)
- 100 ☐ Pain pills (Demerol, codeine, morphine, etc.)
- 101 ☐ Antihistamines or allergy pills

DO YOU NOW DRINK ANY ALCOHOLIC BEVERAGES (BEER, WINE, WHISKEY, GIN, VODKA, ETC)?

102 ☐ No   103 ☐ Yes   IF YES, MARK THE ONE CORRECT ANSWER:

I drink:

- 104 ☐ 2 or less drinks per week.
- 105 ☐ 3 to 6 drinks per week.
- 282 ☐ 7 to 14 drinks per week.
- 275 ☐ 15 to 24 drinks per week.
- 107 ☐ 25 to 40 drinks per week.
- 108 ☐ More than 40 drinks per week.

DID YOU FORMERLY DRINK ANY ALCOHOLIC BEVERAGES (BEER, WINE, WHISKEY, GIN, VODKA, ETC.) AND NO LONGER DO?

109 ☐ No   110 ☐ Yes   IF YES, MARK THE ONE CORRECT ANSWER:

YOUR OWN HEALTH PROFILE: Computer-Assisted

I drank:

- 111 ☐ 2 or less drinks per week.
- 112 ☐ 3 to 6 drinks per week.
- 283 ☐ 7 to 14 drinks per week.
- 276 ☐ 15 to 24 drinks per week.
- 114 ☐ 25 to 40 drinks per week.
- 115 ☐ More than 40 drinks per week.

HAVE YOU EVER BEEN TOLD YOU HAD LIVER DISEASE DUE TO DRINKING?
277 ☐ No   278 ☐ Yes

HAS ANYONE IN YOUR IMMEDIATE FAMILY (PARENTS, BROTHERS, SISTERS) TAKEN HIS OR HER OWN LIFE (COMMITTED SUICIDE)?
116 ☐ No   117 ☐ Yes

DO YOU NOW HAVE OR HAVE YOU HAD FEELINGS THAT LIFE IS NOT WORTH LIVING?
118 ☐ No   119 ☐ Yes

DOES EACH DAY LOOK SO DULL THAT YOU WOULD RATHER NOT WAKE UP IN THE MORNING?
120 ☐ No   121 ☐ Yes

DO YOU WORRY OR FEEL BLUE MUCH OF THE TIME?
122 ☐ No   123 ☐ Yes

DO YOU EVER FEEL LIKE SWEARING?
124 ☐ No   125 ☐ Yes

DO YOU HAVE TROUBLE WITH WAKING UP TOO EARLY OR BEING UNABLE TO STAY ASLEEP?
126 ☐ No   127 ☐ Yes

IF YOU HAD YOUR LIFE TO LIVE OVER AGAIN, WOULD YOU DO MOST EVERYTHING SOME OTHER WAY?
128 ☐ No   129 ☐ Yes

CONCERNING THE FUTURE, DO YOU FEEL SURE, POSITIVE, AND HOPEFUL?
284 ☐ No   285 ☐ Yes

IF YOU WERE SURE YOU COULD GET AWAY WITH IT, WOULD YOU GO INTO A BALL GAME OR THEATER WITHOUT PAYING?
132 ☐ No   133 ☐ Yes

DO YOU FEEL WORTHLESS AND THAT OTHERS WOULD BE BETTER OFF IF YOU WERE DEAD?
134 ☐ No   135 ☐ Yes

DO YOU LIKE EVERYONE YOU KNOW?
136 ☐ No   137 ☐ Yes

HAVE YOU EVER SERIOUSLY CONSIDERED KILLING YOURSELF?
138 ☐ No   139 ☐ Yes

DO YOU GET ANGRY SOMETIMES?
140 ☐ No   141 ☐ Yes

DO YOU OFTEN FEEL ALONE AND LONELY EVEN WHEN THERE ARE OTHERS AROUND YOU?
142 ☐ No   143 ☐ Yes

HAVE YOU LOST YOUR APPETITE OR HAVE YOU HAD VERY MUCH LESS DESIRE TO EAT?
144 ☐ No   145 ☐ Yes

DO YOU SOMETIMES HAVE THOUGHTS TOO BAD TO TELL OTHERS?
146 ☐ No   147 ☐ Yes

YOUR OWN HEALTH PROFILE: Computer-Assisted

DO YOU ENJOY A LITTLE FLIRTING?
148 ☐ No 149 ☐ Yes

DO YOU FEEL DEPRESSED OFTEN (MORE THAN 50% OF THE TIME)?
150 ☐ No 151 ☐ Yes

DO YOU CARRY A GUN OR KNIFE OTHER THAN A POCKET KNIFE? (THIS INCLUDES CARRYING A WEAPON IN YOUR WORK.)
152 ☐ No 153 ☐ Yes

HAVE YOU EVER BEEN ARRESTED FOR A SERIOUS CRIME LIKE ROBBERY OR ATTACKING SOMEONE?
154 ☐ No 155 ☐ Yes

DO YOU THINK HOW YOU LIVE (YOUR ECONOMIC AND SOCIAL STATUS) IS:
156 ☐ Low 157 ☐ Medium 158 ☐ High

HAVE YOU EVER HAD CANCER OR A MALIGNANT TUMOR?
159 ☐ No 160 ☐ Yes
IF YES, MARK WHERE THE CANCER OR MALIGNANT TUMOR WAS LOCATED:

161 ☐ Throat
162 ☐ Colon-Intestines (large bowel)
163 ☐ Breast
164 ☐ Brain or Nervous System
165 ☐ Lung
166 ☐ Rectum
279 ☐ Other (Explain)

167 ☐ Stomach
168 ☐ Hodgkins Disease or Lymphosarcoma
170 ☐ Leukemia
172 ☐ Prostate
173 ☐ Esophagus (swallowing tube)
171 ☐ Ovaries

FOR WOMEN ONLY

HAS YOUR MOTHER OR SISTER HAD BREAST CANCER?
174 ☐ No   175 ☐ Yes

DO YOU EXAMINE YOUR BREASTS EACH MONTH TO DETECT CANCER?
176 ☐ No   177 ☐ Yes

DO YOU GO TO THE DOCTOR FOR A BREAST EXAMINATION AT LEAST ONCE EACH YEAR?
178 ☐ No   179 ☐ Yes

DO YOU HAVE X-RAYS OF YOUR BREASTS (NOT CHEST X-RAYS) FOR CANCER AT LEASE ONCE A YEAR?
180 ☐ No   181 ☐ Yes

HAS YOUR UTERUS (WOMB) BEEN REMOVED?
182 ☐ No   183 ☐ Yes   IF YES, WAS IT REMOVED FOR CANCER?
184 ☐ No   185 ☐ Yes

HAS YOUR CERVIX (NECK OF WOMB) BEEN REMOVED?
186 ☐ No   187 ☐ Yes   IF YES, WAS IT REMOVED FOR CANCER?
188 ☐ No   189 ☐ Yes

HAVE BOTH YOUR OVARIES (SEX GLANDS) BEEN REMOVED?
190 ☐ No   191 ☐ Yes   IF YES, MARK AGE REMOVED
Age removed: 192 _____ years.

DO YOU HAVE VAGINAL BLEEDING (BLEEDING FROM YOUR FEMALES, BIRTH CANAL)?
193 ☐ No   194 ☐ Yes   IF YES, MARK ALL CORRECT ANSWERS ABOUT WHEN THE BLEEDING HAPPENS:
195 ☐ Between menstrual periods.
196 ☐ During or after sexual intercourse.
197 ☐ My periods have stopped, but I still have bleeding once in a while.

YOUR OWN HEALTH PROFILE: Computer-Assisted

- 198 ☐ I am taking female hormones (estrogens) and I only bleed when I am off these hormones.
- 199 ☐ I am taking female hormones (estrogens) but I bleed whether I am taking them or not.
- 226 ☐ Only with my menstrual periods.

HAVE YOU EVER HAD SEXUAL INTERCOURSE?

200 ☐ No   20- ☐ Yes   **IF YES, MARK WHEN IT BEGAN:**

- 202 ☐ Before 20 years old
- 203 ☐ Between 20 and 25 years old
- 204 ☐ After 25 years old

DO YOU NOW TAKE BIRTH CONTROL PILLS?

280 ☐ No   28- ☐ Yes

ARE YOU JEWISH? (CANCER OF THE CERVIX IS VERY RARE IN JEWISH WOMEN)

205 ☐ No   206 ☐ Yes

HAVE YOU EVER HAD A PAP (CANCER) SMEAR?

207 ☐ No   208 ☐ Yes   **IF YES, MARK ALL CORRECT ANSWERS:**

- 209 ☐ Some were not normal in the past 5 years.
- 210 ☐ Three or more were normal in the last 5 years.
- 211 ☐ One was normal within the last 12 months (none not normal).
- 212 ☐ One was normal within the last 5 years (none not normal).
- 213 ☐ I don't know the results.
- 214 ☐ I have not had a pap smear in 5 years.

215

THE LONGEVITY FACTOR

Complete as much of the following information as possible. The more information we have, the more meaningful the report will be. Fill out the name only if you want the name to appear on the report. If the name is not completed, only the first two letters of the last name will print. Your doctor may be able to provide you with some of this information.

NAME _____ _____
(OPTIONAL)   (LAST)   (FIRST)

*BLOOD PRESSURE   SYS   DIA   SYS   DIA
 CURRENT   [   ] [   ]   [   ] [   ]
                                HIGHEST (if available)

*CHOLESTEROL
 CURRENT   [   ] MG%   [   ] MG%
                                HIGHEST (if available)

*TRIGLYCERIDES   [   ] MG%   [   ] MG%
                                HIGHEST (if available)

GLUCOSE 1 HOUR (if available) [   ] MG%   GLUCOSE FASTING (if available) [   ] MG%

YOUR OWN HEALTH PROFILE: Computer-Assisted

KNOWN DIABETIC .... NO ☐ YES ☐

CONTROLLED DIABETIC .... NO ☐ YES ☐

ABNORMAL ELECTROCARDIOGRAM (ECG)
WITHIN LAST THREE YEARS .... NO ☐ YES ☐

FORCED EXPIRATORY VOLUME (1 SECOND)
LESS THAN 60% OF NORMAL .... NO ☐ YES ☐

HISTORY OF HEART ATTACK OR
CORONARY OR ANGINA .... NO ☐ YES ☐

HISTORY OF STROKE .... NO ☐ YES ☐

ABNORMAL SGOT OR SGPT (LIVER TESTS) .... NO ☐ YES ☐

*This information is of special significance and should be supplied whenever possible. If not, average values will be used.

For many people, the best way to get a computerized health profile is through a community group such as a weight loss club or an antismoking clinic. The group doesn't necessarily have to have anything to do with medicine or health. All you need is an efficient director who will get in touch with one of the data processing centers. On the West Coast, for example, numerous Methodist churches have sponsored profiling projects for their congregations, bringing in experts to explain the idea, even providing nurses to take blood samples. Quite a few YMCAs also offer profiling, as do a number of unions, ranging from carpenters' locals to the Screen Actors' Guild.

Health profiling is also beginning to be common in educational institutions in the United States. At some colleges it is part of basic medical services for entering freshmen; at others it has become a unit of study in health classes. One audacious high school teacher assigned her students the task of profiling their own parents.

Increasingly government is getting involved. The air force has taken up profiling in an attempt to prevent heart disease among its personnel, and HEW, at its Center for Disease Control in Atlanta, has incorporated the technique into its employee health plan. In Canada, nearly 18,000 civil servants in the city of Ottawa have been profiled, and health questionnaires (see page 198) have also been sent to all Canadians receiving social security. Industry is an ideal place to practice preventive medicine, says Dr. Edgar Brethauer, Jr., for the forthright reason that "prevention improves production." Chief physician at ALCOA's headquarters in Pittsburgh, Dr. Brethauer administers health profiles as part of the periodic medical checkups given to employees. One particularly vivid memory is of an executive who came to Brethauer's office to get his profile printout. The man opened the envelope, sat down, and read his profile. Then he rose, pulled out the pack of cigarettes from his pocket, and without a word dropped it into Brethauer's wastebasket. Says Dr. Brethauer, "That single sheet of paper predicted he would lose four years of life if he went on smoking"; the man has not smoked again. Other corporations using profiling today include Ford Motor Company, Sears Roebuck, Sentry Insurance, and Kimberly Clark, the paper company, which not only profiles its employees, but has provided them with a $2.5 million health center and gym to help them alter their risks.

How does group profiling work? Here, to end this chapter, is an example showing the way one small company went about it—Superior Farms of Bakersfield, California, subsidiary of the Superior Oil Company.

Two summers ago, in the air-conditioned meeting room of a Bakersfield motel, eighty Californians got together one morning. They were casually dressed and had the easy manner of people who work the land, although they varied in racial type from swarthy *Mexicanos* to sandy-haired young *Anglo* university graduates.

The men were farmers, all of them, field superintendents. Their boss was present too, Fred W. Andrew, erect, barrel chested, and the tallest man in the room, even sitting down, as he was, in the back row, like a junior high school teacher with his students at assembly.

Backed by an oil company, Andrew had created the farm subsidiary in just six years, skillfully building the staff to make it prosper. The whole enterprise includes more than 37,000 acres in separate parcels extending from Palm Springs to Tucson, Arizona, annually lavishing thousands of tons of fertilizers, millions of gallons of pesticides, and whole rivers of irrigation water to grow year-round harvests of grapes and peaches, potatoes and melons, plums and pistachios, figs, cucumbers, alfalfa, olives, apricots—thirty-two different crops in all, most of them shipped east for profit.

About the staff that superintended the operation, Andrew said: "I've gone through a lot of men, including plenty of slack ones who either left or got booted out. The good ones I've taken great pains to hold on to. This is a team that knows how to perform.

"Now I'm worried about them. A lot of them started as field hands. Today they supervise hundreds of employees, but they're still eating and living as if they did hard physical labor, and I think it's ruining their health." This was why Andrew had contacted Interhealth, the San Diego profiling center.

So a few weeks earlier, Interhealth had sent a crew of nurses to Bakersfield to take the farmers' blood samples, check their blood pressure, and get them to fill out health profile questionnaires, which were then brought to San Diego to be run through the computer.

Back with the results today was Dr. Charles M. Ross of Interhealth, past president of the Society of Prospective Medicine. Ross regularly travels up, down, and across the continent, analyzing and exhorting such diverse groups as Harvard clubs, government employees, college students, and the elderly inhabitants of Leisure Worlds. These were the first farmers he had faced. Dark haired and trimly built, he looked almost frail next to Fred Andrew; but in fact Ross is a walking testimonial to the preventive medicine life. At the time of his Bakersfield visit he was 51 years of age, but his medical risk age was only 42.

With an audience, Ross comes on at first as merely mild and friendly. Then, gradually, his voice warms and deepens into eloquence, until soon the audience is very quiet, just listening. This is what happened in the motel at Bakersfield.

YOUR OWN HEALTH PROFILE: Computer-Assisted

Ross's message for the farmers that day was not a reassuring one. In groups as large as eighty people there will always be some high health risks, but usually they are canceled out by equally low risks, yielding an average risk age that is within a month or two of the average chronological age. This was not true at Bakersfield, where the chronological average age was 39.8, the average risk age 40.8, a gap of a full year, and the highest average deficit Ross had seen in any group with which he had worked. On the optimistic side, the potential for reduction was large too—4.2 years, down to an average risk age of 36.6.

Diagnosis delivered, Ross went on to speak of the rest of the American population. Since 1900, infectious diseases, he explained, have been all but wiped out as causes of death in the United States, but this decline has been offset by a dramatic rise in heart disease, cancer, strokes, and accidents. Onto a projection screen he flashed a graph showing the U.S. death rate, a line that since 1950 reads almost completely flat. Ross glanced at the faces in the rows before him. He said, "You don't let farm machinery get in such bad shape that you have to spend all your time repairing it. Yet that's what we have been doing with our health care. First we let people fall apart, then we try putting them back together again with money. It doesn't work.

"Last year the United States spent $140 billion on the treatment of disease—and with a net lack of effect on the death rate. I think it should be apparent to all of us, the government included, that we've got to try something different."

Then he got more personal again. He had an assistant pass out the individual health profile printouts, and each member of the gathering studied his own report while Ross explained the differing risks. How obesity can lead to high blood pressure, and how high blood pressure in turn increases the chances for an early stroke. How 50 percent of automobile fatalities involve alcohol, and 11 percent marijuana.

There was a break for the motel luncheon—a buffet decidedly high in cholesterol, as Ross pointed out wryly—and then the physician went back to the podium to describe ways of cutting risks. He talked especially about diet and exercise, because these were major problems for the Bakersfield group. After an hour of that, he answered questions from the audience for another hour. Then he consulted individually with people whose risks were particularly high. When Ross finally left for the little Bakersfield airport it was late afternoon, and he bore with him a crate of newly picked grapes and another of peaches, gifts from the appreciative farmers. As for the farmers themselves, they were left not only with a message to think about, but something in their hands to study and reflect upon: their health profiles.

17
YOUR OWN HEALTH PROFILE: Do It Yourself

This system is derived, with permission, from the Health Hazard Appraisal techniques outlined by doctors Lewis Robbins and Jack Hall in their book for physicians, *How to Practice Prospective Medicine*. To make it a little easier to use, our adaptation is not quite so individualized or precise as the Robbins-Hall model, but it will give you a picture of where you stand medically that is both broad and detailed, summed up in a medical risk age that may vary considerably from your chronological one. All you need is a couple of sharp pencils and, if available, one of those little pocket calculators you usually save for doing your income tax—plus about an hour of free time.

Before beginning, we should point out several things. First, you will be working with a numerical system consisting of *advantage points* and *disadvantage points*. In all cases, these points express the extent of your personal, individual risk, as compared with the risk of the average person in your age-sex-race category.

The lower you score on each item, the better. *Disadvantage points* are all larger than 1.0, signifying a relatively high risk. In contrast, *advantage points* are limited to 1.0 or below, signifying risks that are relatively low; 1.0 itself signifies precisely average—not necessarily a state of optimum health, incidentally. The average middle-aged American, for example, is about 15 pounds overweight when compared to optimum weight charts.

A second preliminary note: The arithmetic you will be asked to perform will not be difficult, but its logic may at times seem a little inexplicable; it is, however, based on long-established actuarial principles.

Directions

To guide you through your calculations, we will set down the arithmetic for a hypothetical person, providing blanks alongside for you to fill in with your own figures as they accrue along the way. Our example will be a healthy male, white, American, in the middle of the age tables—37 years old. Call him "John." On the following pages, health indicators to consider are on the left-hand page; John's figures are in the first column on the right-hand page; and the second column is for your entries.

First, turn to the mortality tables printed on pages 39 to 52 and find the list of ten-year causes of death that applies to you. John's list for himself, as a white, 37-year-old male, is shown in the first column on the top of the next page. In the second column is a blank list for you to fill in.

YOUR OWN HEALTH PROFILE: Do It Yourself

JOHN'S RISK LIST	YOUR OWN RISK LIST
1. Arteriosclerotic heart disease	1.
2. Motor vehicle accidents	2.
3. Suicide	3.
4. Cirrhosis of the liver	4.
5. Homicide	5.
6. Lung cancer	6.
7. Stroke	7.
8. Pneumonia	8.
9. Cancer of the large intestine and rectum	9.
10. Brain cancer	10.

On the following pages you will be going down this list of causes of death, and, one by one, will compute your individual risks, as compared with the average for your category. Follow John's example for method, and circle the number appropriate to you.

John's list of risks is headed by arteriosclerotic heart disease, the most common cause of death among Americans, male or female. Because this disease involves so many risk indicators (family history, smoking, exercise, weight, diabetes, blood pressure, cholesterol), it is by far the most complicated to compute. Once you finish this one, the others will be easy.

1. ARTERIOSCLEROTIC HEART DISEASE

a. Family history

Both parents died of heart disease before age 60

One parent died of heart disease before age 60

Parents survive (i.e., neither has suffered fatal heart disease) and both are still under 60

Neither parent died of heart disease before 60

b. Smoking

More than ½ pack of cigarettes a day

Less than ½ pack of cigarettes a day (but do smoke)

Stopped smoking within past 7 years

Stopped smoking 10 or more years ago

c. Exercise (4 times per week, on the average)

Less than ½ mile walked, or under 5 flights of stairs climbed, or equivalent

½ to 1½ miles, or 5 to 15 flights, or equivalent

1½ to 2 miles, or 15 to 20 flights, or equivalent

More than the above

YOUR OWN HEALTH PROFILE: Do It Yourself

JOHN'S SCORE		YOUR SCORE	
ADVANTAGE POINTS	DISADVANTAGE POINTS	ADVANTAGE POINTS	DISADVANTAGE POINTS
	1.4		1.4
	(1.2)		1.2
1.0		1.0	
.9		.9	

In John's case, his mother died of heart disease at age 56, so he circles the disadvantage point 1.2 as his score for this factor.		Circle the appropriate score for you.	
	1.5		1.5
	(1.1)		1.1
.7		.7	
.5		.5	
John circles his score.		Circle yours.	
	2.5		2.5
(1.0)		1.0	
.6		.6	
.5		.5	
		Again, circle score and proceed onward.	

227

THE LONGEVITY FACTOR

ARTERIOSCLEROTIC HEART DISEASE (cont.)

d. Weight

75% overweight _____

50% overweight _____

15% overweight _____

10% underweight _____

Use the weight tables in Appendix A to figure your score; then circle it.

e. Cholesterol

280 or above _____

220 _____

180 _____

If you do not know your cholesterol level, give yourself the benefit of the doubt and circle the average figure, which is 1.0 advantage point.

f. Diabetes

Yes, I have been diagnosed as diabetic, but am not under medical treatment _____

Yes, but I am being treated _____

No _____

228

YOUR OWN HEALTH PROFILE: Do It Yourself

JOHN'S SCORE		YOUR SCORE	
ADVANTAGE POINTS	DISADVANTAGE POINTS	ADVANTAGE POINTS	DISADVANTAGE POINTS
	2.5		2.5
	1.5		1.5
(1.0)		1.0	
.8		.8	

Circle your score.

	1.6		1.6
1.0		1.0	
.5		.5	

Circle your score.

	3.0		3.0
	2.5		2.5
(1.0)		1.0	

Circle your score.

THE LONGEVITY FACTOR

ARTERIOSCLEROTIC HEART DISEASE (cont.)

g. Blood pressure

If you do not know what your blood pressure is, use the average figure, a single 1.0 advantage point. If you do know, use the sets of readings, systolic and diastolic, below. In figuring your score, use the single higher of the two readings unless both score more than 1.0. If both score more than 1.0, circle them both for computation.

Systolic blood pressure (when your heart is pumping)

200	
180	
160	
140	
120	

Diastolic blood pressure (when your heart is at rest)

106	
100	
94	
88	
82	

YOUR OWN HEALTH PROFILE: Do It Yourself

JOHN'S SCORE		YOUR SCORE	
ADVANTAGE POINTS	DISADVANTAGE POINTS	ADVANTAGE POINTS	DISADVANTAGE POINTS
	3.2		3.2
	2.2		2.2
	(1.4)		1.4
.8		.8	
.4		.4	
	4.0		4.0
	2.2		2.2
	1.3		1.3
.8		.8	
.4		.4	

John's blood pressure is 160 systolic over 85 diastolic. Therefore, he circles the systolic, because it scores 1.4, and ignores the diastolic, since it scores only .8.

Circle your score.

ARTERIOSCLEROTIC HEART DISEASE (cont.)

You have now covered all the separate factors affecting arteriosclerotic heart disease. Before combining them into one overall risk rating, list the figures compactly, so they will be easily available during computation.

a. Family history _____
b. Smoking _____
c. Exercise _____
d. Weight _____
e. Cholesterol _____
f. Diabetes _____
g. Blood pressure _____

Next, compute your overall risk factor for arteriosclerotic heart disease by the method described in the box below. Once again, John serves as an example:

METHOD	SAMPLE COMPUTATION
1. First, figure the disadvantage point subtotal:	
a. Add up the disadvantage points.	Family history 1.2 Smoking 1.1 Cholesterol 1.6 Blood pressure 1.4 5.3
b. From this, subtract the number of separate disadvantage points.	−4.0
c. This number is the disadvantage point subtotal.	1.3

YOUR OWN HEALTH PROFILE: Do It Yourself

JOHN'S SUMMARY		YOUR SUMMARY	
ADVANTAGE POINTS	DISADVANTAGE POINTS	ADVANTAGE POINTS	DISADVANTAGE POINTS
	1.2		
	1.1		
1.0			
1.0			
	1.6		
1.0			
	1.4		

2. Then figure the advantage point subtotal:
   a. Multiply all the advantage points by one another.

   Exercise 1.0
   Weight 1.0
   Diabetes 1.0
   (1.0) × (1.0) × (1.0) = 1.0

   b. If necessary, round off to one decimal. This is the advantage point subtotal. Subtotal 1.0

3. Then add up the two subtotals:

   Disadvantage subtotal 1.3
   Advantage subtotal 1.0
   2.3

4. And, if there are only disadvantage points, with no advantage points, add one point (1.0) penalty: + Penalty ____

This total is the composite risk factor for this one disease: 2.3

THE LONGEVITY FACTOR

ARTERIOSCLEROTIC HEART DISEASE (cont.)

Now it's time to figure your own composite risk factor for arteriosclerotic heart disease. To help you with your calculations, we will repeat John's figures; you may also refer back to the box on the previous page to renew instructions. You'll soon get into the swing of it.

John has both advantage points and disadvantage points for arteriosclerotic heart disease.

JOHN'S SCORE		YOUR SCORE
First he adds up his disadvantage points:		Add your disadvantage points:
Family history	1.2	
Smoking	1.1	
Cholesterol	1.6	
Blood pressure	1.4	
	5.3	
Then, because there are four separate categories in which he scored disadvantage points, he subtracts 4:		Subtract the number of your disadvantage categories:
	−4.0	
Subtotal	1.3	
Then he multiplies all his advantage points (exercise, weight, and absence of diabetes) one by the other:		Multiply your advantage points:
1.0 × 1.0 × 1.0 = subtotal, 1.0		

234

YOUR OWN HEALTH PROFILE: Do It Yourself

JOHN'S SCORE	YOUR SCORE

Then the subtotals are combined:
 	
      1.3
    +1.0
      2.3
 	
John has advantage points as well as disadvantage points, so he need not add a penalty point.
 	
John's overall risk factor for death from arteriosclerotic heart disease is <u>2.3</u>
	Combine your subtotals:
	
	If you have only disadvantage points, add a penalty of 1.0.
	
	YOUR OWN RISK FACTOR FOR ARTERIOSCLEROTIC HEART DISEASE IS _____.

THE LONGEVITY FACTOR

2. MOTOR VEHICLE ACCIDENTS

Pass on now to the second highest risk of death for your age group. In John's case, this is motor vehicle accidents, with just three contributing factors to consider—drinking habits, mileage per year, and seat belt use.

a. Drinking

    More than 40 drinks per week (1 drink = 1 glass of wine or beer, or 1½ ounces of hard liquor) _____

    25 to 40 drinks per week _____

    15 to 24 drinks per week _____

    Less than 15 drinks per week _____

    Nondrinker _____

b. Mileage per year

    Figure out the total number of miles you drive (or are driven) annually, and divide it by 10,000. If the result is 1.0 or less, enter it under advantage points; if more, under disadvantage points.

c. Use of seat or shoulder belt

    Less than 10% of time (as either driver or passenger) _____

    10 to 25% of time _____

    25 to 75% of time _____

    75 to 100% of time _____

YOUR OWN HEALTH PROFILE: Do It Yourself

JOHN'S SCORE		YOUR SCORE	
ADVANTAGE POINTS	DISADVANTAGE POINTS	ADVANTAGE POINTS	DISADVANTAGE POINTS
	12.5		12.5
	5.0		5.0
	(2.0)		2.0
1.0		1.0	
.5		.5	

Circle your score.

	(3.5)		
(John drives 35,000 miles per year)		**Insert and circle your score.**	
	1.1		1.1
(1.0)		1.0	
.9		.9	
.8		.8	

Circle your score.

THE LONGEVITY FACTOR

MOTOR VEHICLE ACCIDENTS (cont.)

Again, summarize your figures for motor vehicle accidents, before figuring your composite risk factor.

    a. Drinking _____

    b. Mileage per year _____

    c. Use of seat or shoulder belt _____

YOUR OWN HEALTH PROFILE: Do It Yourself

John's Summary		Your Summary	
ADVANTAGE POINTS	DISADVANTAGE POINTS	ADVANTAGE POINTS	DISADVANTAGE POINTS
	2.0		
	3.5		
1.0			

Again, John has a mixed bag of advantage points and disadvantage points. First he adds up his disadvantage points:	Figure your composite risk, filling it in below. If you have only disadvantage points, don't forget to add the penalty point.
Drinking 2.0 Mileage per year 3.5 Total 5.5 Then he subtracts his number of disadvantage categories: −2.0 3.5 The advantage point subtotal is a single 1.0. It is added: +1.0 4.5 John's overall risk factor for death from motor vehicle accidents is **4.5.**	YOUR OWN RISK FACTOR FOR MOTOR VEHICLE ACCIDENTS IS _____.

3. SUICIDE

The next of John's risks is suicide, a relatively simple calculation based on three conditions:

a. Depression

        Often depressed _____

        Seldom depressed _____

b. Family history of suicide
(parents, grandparents, sisters, brothers)

        Yes _____

        No _____

c. Drinking

        40 or more drinks per week _____

        Less than 40 drinks per week _____

Summary:

    a. Depression _____

    b. Family history of suicide _____

    c. Drinking _____

YOUR OWN HEALTH PROFILE: Do It Yourself

JOHN'S SCORE		YOUR SCORE	
ADVANTAGE POINTS	DISADVANTAGE POINTS	ADVANTAGE POINTS	DISADVANTAGE POINTS
	2.5		2.5
(1.0)	1.0		1.0
		Circle your score.	
	2.5		2.5
(1.0)	1.0		1.0
		Circle your score.	
	2.5		2.5
(1.0)	1.0		1.0
		Circle your score.	

John's Summary   **Your Summary**

1.0
1.0
1.0

John has only advantage points.

Follow through with your figures, adding a penalty point if needed.

He multiplies his advantage points:

$1.0 \times 1.0 \times 1.0 = 1.0$

John's overall risk factor for death from suicide is <u>1.0</u>.

YOUR OWN RISK FACTOR FOR SUICIDE IS _____.

4. CIRRHOSIS OF THE LIVER

The next risk for John is cirrhosis of the liver. The questions regarding drinking, you will notice, are a little more searching here than for suicide.

a. Drinking

More than 40 drinks per week	_____
25 to 40 drinks a week, and you sometimes get drunk	_____
15 to 24 drinks per week but never drunk	_____
7 to 14 drinks per week	_____
Less than 7 drinks per week	_____
Stopped drinking before any signs of cirrhosis appeared	_____
Nondrinker	_____

YOUR OWN HEALTH PROFILE: Do It Yourself

JOHN'S SCORE		YOUR SCORE	
ADVANTAGE POINTS	DISADVANTAGE POINTS	ADVANTAGE POINTS	DISADVANTAGE POINTS
	12.5		12.5
	5.0		5.0
	(2.0)		2.0
1.0		1.0	
.2		.2	
.2		.2	
.1		.1	

Circle your score.

No summary is necessary because you are dealing with a single advantage or disadvantage point.

John subtracts the number of categories from the total of his disadvantage points: 2.0 $\underline{-1.0}$ 1.0 Because he scores only in the disadvantage column, he adds a penalty point of 1.0: 1.0 $\underline{+1.0}$ 2.0 John's overall risk factor for death from cirrhosis is **2.0**.	Calculate your score. YOUR OWN RISK FACTOR FOR CIRRHOSIS IS _____.

5. HOMICIDE

John's risk number 5 is homicide, affected by these considerations:

a. Have you ever been arrested for assault?

        Yes _____

        No _____

b. Do you often carry a weapon (either on your job or off)?

        Yes _____

        No _____

c. Do you consume 40 or more drinks per week?

        Yes _____

        No _____

Summary:

    a. Arrest record _____

    b. Weapon _____

    c. Drinking _____

YOUR OWN HEALTH PROFILE: Do It Yourself

JOHN'S SCORE		YOUR SCORE	
ADVANTAGE POINTS	DISADVANTAGE POINTS	ADVANTAGE POINTS	DISADVANTAGE POINTS
	10.0		10.0
(1.0)		1.0	
		Circle your score.	
	2.0		2.0
(1.0)		1.0	
		Circle your score.	
	2.5		2.5
(1.0)		1.0	
		Circle your score.	
John's Summary		**Your Summary**	
1.0			
1.0			
1.0			

John multiplies the advantage points.

$1.0 \times 1.0 \times 1.0 = 1.0$

John's overall risk factor for death from homicide is 1.0.

Calculate yours, adding a penalty point, if needed.

YOUR OWN RISK FACTOR FOR HOMICIDE IS _____.

THE LONGEVITY FACTOR

6. LUNG CANCER

Sixth on John's risk list is lung cancer, a disease that has moved several notches up the list for male deaths in the past twenty years and is now moving fast up the female list.

a. Daily consumption of cigarettes

        2 packs or more

        1 pack

        ½ pack

        Less than ½ pack, but do smoke

b. Never smoked habitually

c. Former smokers should calculate as follows: take the amount you *used* to smoke, reduce it by 20%, then reduce it by an additional 10% for each year since you quit—but do not allow your score to fall below .2.

YOUR OWN HEALTH PROFILE: Do It Yourself

JOHN'S SCORE		YOUR SCORE	
ADVANTAGE POINTS	DISADVANTAGE POINTS	ADVANTAGE POINTS	DISADVANTAGE POINTS
	2.0		2.0
	1.5		1.5
	(1.1)		1.1
.8		.8	
.2		.2	

Circle your score.

John's score for the ½ pack he smokes daily is 1.1 disadvantage points.

He subtracts the number of categories from his total:

    1.1
 −1.0
     .1

And adds one penalty point:

 +1.0
    1.1

John's overall risk factor for death from lung cancer is **1.1**.

Your calculation (including penalty point, if needed):

YOUR OWN RISK FACTOR FOR LUNG CANCER IS _____.

247

7. STROKE

The next in order of John's risks is stroke—vascular lesions affecting the central nervous system. The preconditions will be familiar from questions already answered about heart disease, but some of the point values differ.

a. Smoking (answer only one)

    Smoke cigarettes _____

    Stopped smoking _____

    Never smoked _____

b. Have you been diagnosed as a diabetic?

    Yes, not controlled _____

    Yes, but controlled _____

    No _____

c. Cholesterol

    280 or above _____

    220 _____

    180 _____

If you do not know your cholesterol level, assume 1.0, average.

YOUR OWN HEALTH PROFILE: Do It Yourself

JOHN'S SCORE

ADVANTAGE POINTS	DISADVANTAGE POINTS
	ⓘ.2
1.0	
.8	
	3.0
	2.5
①.0	
	①.6
1.0	
.5	

YOUR SCORE

ADVANTAGE POINTS	DISADVANTAGE POINTS
	1.2
1.0	
.8	
Circle your score.	
	3.0
	2.5
1.0	
Circle your score.	
	1.6
1.0	
.5	
Circle your score.	

THE LONGEVITY FACTOR

STROKE (cont.)

d. Blood pressure

If you do not know what your blood pressure is, use the average figure, a single 1.0 advantage point. If you do know, use the sets of readings, systolic and diastolic, below. In figuring your score, use the single higher of the two readings unless both score more than 1.0. If both score more than 1.0, circle them both for computation.

Systolic

200	
180	
160	
140	
120	

Diastolic

106	
100	
94	
88	
82	

YOUR OWN HEALTH PROFILE: Do It Yourself

JOHN'S SCORE		YOUR SCORE	
ADVANTAGE POINTS	DISADVANTAGE POINTS	ADVANTAGE POINTS	DISADVANTAGE POINTS
	3.2		3.2
	2.2		2.2
	(1.4)		1.4
.8		.8	
.4		.4	
		Circle your score.	
	4.0		4.0
	2.2		2.2
	1.3		1.3
.8		.8	
.4		.4	
		Circle your score.	

STROKE (cont.)

Summary:
- a. Smoking
- b. Diabetes
- c. Cholesterol
- d. Blood pressure

YOUR OWN HEALTH PROFILE: Do It Yourself

John's Summary	Your Summary
1.2	
1.0	
1.6	
1.4	

John has a mix of advantage and disadvantage points.

Your calculation (including penalty point, if needed):

He adds the disadvantage points:

Smoking	1.2
Cholesterol	1.6
Blood pressure	1.4
	4.2

He subtracts the number of disadvantage categories:

```
  4.2
 -3.0
  1.2
```

He multiplies the advantage points; having only one, his subtotal is:

```
  1.0
```

He adds the two subtotals:

```
   1.0
  +1.2
   2.2
```

John's overall risk factor for death from stroke is **2.2**.

YOUR OWN RISK FACTOR FOR STROKE IS _____.

253

8. PNEUMONIA

John's risk number 8 is pneumonia. Preconditions:

a. Drinking

    Averaging more than 40 drinks per week _____

    Averaging less than 40 drinks per week _____

    Nondrinker _____

b. History of bacterial pneumonia

    Yes _____

    No _____

c. Symptoms of emphysema

    Yes _____

    No _____

d. Smoking

    Over ½ pack a day _____

    ½ pack or less a day _____

Summary:

    a. Drinking _____

    b. History of bacterial pneumonia _____

    c. Symptoms of emphysema _____

    d. Smoking _____

All John's points are advantages.

YOUR OWN HEALTH PROFILE: Do It Yourself

JOHN'S SCORE		YOUR SCORE	
ADVANTAGE POINTS	DISADVANTAGE POINTS	ADVANTAGE POINTS	DISADVANTAGE POINTS
	3.0		3.0
(1.0)			1.0
1.0			1.0
		Circle your score.	
	2.0		2.0
(1.0)			1.0
		Circle your score.	
	2.0		2.0
(1.0)			1.0
		Circle your score.	
	1.2		1.2
(1.0)			1.0
John's Summary		**Your Summary**	
1.0			
1.0			
1.0			
1.0			

He multiplies his points:

$1.0 \times 1.0 \times 1.0 \times 1.0 = 1.0$

John's overall risk factor for death from pneumonia is 1.0.

Your calculation (including penalty point, if applicable):

YOUR OWN RISK FACTOR FOR PNEUMONIA IS _____.

9. CANCER OF THE LARGE INTESTINE AND RECTUM

John's risk number 9 is cancer of the large intestine and rectum. Preconditions:

a. Have polyps been observed in your intestine or rectum during a proctological examination?

    Yes _____

    No _____

b. Have you had rectal bleeding, but not sought a medical diagnosis?

    Yes _____

    No _____

c. Have you suffered from ulcerative colitis?

    Yes, for 10 years or more _____

    Yes, for less than 10 years _____

    No _____

d. If you have an annual sigmoidoscopy (examination of the rectum and lower intestine with a lighted instrument), multiply the total of the above points by .3 and enter here (in the advantage column if 1.0 or less, in the disadvantage column if greater than 1.0).

Summary:

    a. Intestinal polyps _____

    b. Rectal bleeding _____

    c. Ulcerative colitis _____

    d. Annual sigmoidoscopy _____

YOUR OWN HEALTH PROFILE: Do It Yourself

JOHN'S SCORE		YOUR SCORE	
ADVANTAGE POINTS	DISADVANTAGE POINTS	ADVANTAGE POINTS	DISADVANTAGE POINTS
	2.5		2.5
(1.0)		1.0	
		Circle your score.	
	3.3		3.3
(1.0)		1.0	
		Circle your score.	
	4.0		4.0
	2.0		2.0
(1.0)		1.0	
		Circle your score.	

John's Summary

1.0
1.0
1.0

All John's points are advantage points.
He multiplies them:

1.0 × 1.0 × 1.0 = 1.0

John's overall risk factor for death from cancer of the large intestine and rectum is <u>1.0</u>.

Your Summary

Your calculation:

YOUR OWN RISK FACTOR FOR CANCER OF THE LARGE INTESTINE AND RECTUM IS _____.

10. BRAIN CANCER

John's risk number 10 is brain cancer. No clear-cut precursors have yet been established for several fairly prominent causes of death, including brain tumor, leukemia, and Hodgkin's disease; it is assumed that personal habits do not affect them (though heredity may). If one of these diseases crops up on your list of health hazards, simply assign yourself an average risk, or 1.0, as John has done here.

This concludes the calculations of separate risks for John, a white male American aged 37.

Almost certainly there will be risks of your own, not shared with John. If you are a woman, these may well include:

- Breast cancer (the leading cause of death in several women's age groups)
- Cancer of the cervix
- Cancer of the uterus

And if your age group is different from John's, your list of causes of death may also differ. Each disease for which a

YOUR OWN HEALTH PROFILE: Do It Yourself

JOHN'S SCORE		YOUR SCORE	
ADVANTAGE POINTS	DISADVANTAGE POINTS	ADVANTAGE POINTS	DISADVANTAGE POINTS
1.0			
John's overall risk factor for death from brain cancer is **1.0**.		YOUR OWN RISK FACTOR FOR BRAIN CANCER IS _____.	

computing formula is given in this chapter causes 1% or more of deaths in the United States yearly. Some major diseases that are not on John's list, but that could be on yours, are:

- Hypertensive heart disease
- Diabetes mellitus
- Diseases of the arteries (other than in the heart or brain)
- Emphysema
- Rheumatic heart disease

On the following pages you will find the figures necessary to compute your risk factor for these diseases.

BREAST CANCER

YOUR SCORE

	ADVANTAGE POINTS	DISADVANTAGE POINTS

Preconditions:

a. Mother or sister suffered breast cancer:

Yes		2.0
No	1.0	

If you score disadvantage points because you answered yes, your risk can be cut by following proper examination procedures—either monthly breast self-examination, or X-ray mammography at regular intervals. If this is the case, enter an advantage point of 1.0, in addition to the disadvantage points, and calculate on the basis of both.

b. Neither mother nor sister suffered breast cancer, and:

1. You fail to follow examination procedures	1.0	
2. You do follow them		.5

Calculate your composite figures, adding a penalty point, if needed.

YOUR RISK FACTOR FOR BREAST CANCER IS _____.

YOUR OWN HEALTH PROFILE: Do It Yourself

CANCER OF THE CERVIX

YOUR SCORE

	ADVANTAGE POINTS	DISADVANTAGE POINTS
Preconditions:		
a. Economic and social status		
Low		2.0
Average	1.0	
High	.5	
b. Jewish parentage (associated with low risk of cervical cancer)		
Yes	.1	
No	1.0	
c. Age of first sexual intercourse		
Teens		3.0
20–25	1.0	
Over 25	.5	

Summary

a. Economic and social status

b. Jewish parentage

c. Age of first sexual intercourse

To get your rating for this disease, calculate the points scored in a, b and c (above) by the usual method, then multiply your result by the answer you provide for d (next page); if applicable.

THE LONGEVITY FACTOR

CANCER OF THE CERVIX (cont.)

YOUR SCORE

ADVANTAGE POINTS	DISADVANTAGE POINTS

d. Pap smear test

Negative Pap test within past 5 years: .7

Negative Pap test within past year: .5

Three negative Pap tests within past 5 years: .1

Calculate:

YOUR RISK FACTOR FOR CANCER OF THE CERVIX IS _____.

CANCER OF THE UTERUS

YOUR SCORE

ADVANTAGE POINTS	DISADVANTAGE POINTS

Preconditions:

Have you had unusual vaginal bleeding, undiagnosed?

| Yes | | 2.0 |
| No | 1.0 | |

Calculate as usual, adding a penalty point, if necessary.

YOUR RISK FACTOR FOR CANCER OF THE UTERUS IS _____.

HYPERTENSIVE HEART DISEASE

YOUR SCORE

	ADVANTAGE POINTS	DISADVANTAGE POINTS

Preconditions:

a. Weight (refer to weight tables, pages 280 to 283)

	ADVANTAGE	DISADVANTAGE
75% overweight		2.5
50% overweight		1.5
15% overweight	1.0	
10% underweight	.8	

b. Blood pressure

If you do not know what your blood pressure is, use the average figure, a single 1.0. If you do know, use the sets of readings, systolic and diastolic, below. In figuring your score, use the higher of the two readings unless both score more than 1.0. If both score more than 1.0, circle them both for computation.

Systolic blood pressure

200		3.2
180		2.2
160		1.4
140	.8	
120	.4	

Diastolic blood pressure

106		3.7
100		2.0
94		1.3
88	.8	
82	.4	

YOUR OWN HEALTH PROFILE: Do It Yourself

YOUR SCORE

ADVANTAGE POINTS   DISADVANTAGE POINTS

Summary

a. Weight _____

b. Blood pressure _____

Calculate, not forgetting the penalty point, if applicable:

YOUR RISK FACTOR FOR HYPERTENSIVE HEART DISEASE IS _____.

THE LONGEVITY FACTOR

DIABETES MELLITUS

YOUR SCORE

	ADVANTAGE POINTS	DISADVANTAGE POINTS

Preconditions:

a. Weight (refer to weight tables, pages 280 to 283)

	ADVANTAGE	DISADVANTAGE
75% overweight		4.0
50% overweight		3.0
30% overweight		1.5
15% overweight	1.0	
At recommended weight, or 10% under	.9	

b. Family history (parents, brothers, sisters): have any suffered from diabetes?

	ADVANTAGE	DISADVANTAGE
Yes		2.6
No	.9	

Summary

a. Weight _____

b. Family history _____

Calculation, including penalty point, if needed:

YOUR RISK FACTOR FOR DIABETES IS _____.

YOUR OWN HEALTH PROFILE: Do It Yourself

DISEASES OF THE ARTERIES
(other than the heart and brain)

	YOUR SCORE	
	ADVANTAGE POINTS	DISADVANTAGE POINTS

Preconditions:

a. Do you smoke?

Yes, cigarettes		1.2
Yes, cigars or a pipe	1.0	
Did smoke, but have quit	1.0	
Never smoked habitually	.8	

b. Are you diabetic?

Yes, and not controlled		3.0
Yes, but controlled		2.5
No	1.0	

c. Cholesterol

280		1.5
220	1.0	
180	.5	

If you don't know your cholesterol level, insert average: 1.0 advantage point.

d. Blood pressure

If you do not know what your blood pressure is, use the average figure, 1.0. If you do know, use the sets of readings, systolic and diastolic, below. In figuring your score, use the higher of the two readings unless both score more than 1.0. If both score more than 1.0, circle them both for computation.

THE LONGEVITY FACTOR

DISEASES OF THE ARTERIES (cont.)

YOUR SCORE

	ADVANTAGE POINTS	DISADVANTAGE POINTS
Systolic		
200		3.1
180		2.1
160		1.3
140	.7	
120	.4	
Diastolic		
106		3.4
100		1.8
94		1.2
88	.7	
82	.4	

Summary

a. Smoking

b. Diabetes

c. Cholesterol

d. Blood pressure

Compute, adding the penalty point, if needed:

YOUR RISK FACTOR FOR DISEASES OF THE ARTERIES IS ____.

YOUR OWN HEALTH PROFILE: Do It Yourself

EMPHYSEMA

YOUR SCORE

ADVANTAGE POINTS   DISADVANTAGE POINTS

Preconditions:

a. Daily cigarette consumption

2 packs or more		2.5
1 pack		1.8
½ pack		1.1
Less than ½ pack, but do smoke	.8	

b. Never smoked habitually   .2

Former smokers should calculate as follows: take the amount you *used* to smoke, and reduce it by 30% for every year since you quit, but do not allow your score to fall below .2.

No summary is necessary because you are dealing with a single advantage or disadvantage point.

Your calculation, including penalty point, if needed:

YOUR RISK FACTOR FOR EMPHYSEMA IS _____.

RHEUMATIC HEART DISEASE

YOUR SCORE

	ADVANTAGE POINTS	DISADVANTAGE POINTS

Preconditions:

Have you ever had a heart murmur for which the cause was not diagnosed, or rheumatic fever that went untreated?

Yes		10.0
No	1.0	

Compute, adding penalty point, if needed:

YOUR RISK FACTOR FOR RHEUMATIC HEART DISEASE IS ____.

YOUR OWN HEALTH PROFILE: Do It Yourself

Now that you have figured your separate risks, put them all together, learning the best (or the worst) about your predicted health in the decade that lies ahead. To guide you through the arithmetic, we shall wheel John back into action. Turn the page.

THE LONGEVITY FACTOR

Below is John's list of potential causes of death, with some figures filled in beside them, which will be explained after you too have once more listed your own risks on the facing page.

JOHN'S SCORE

	A DEATHS PER 100,000	×	B JOHN'S INDIVIDUAL RISK FACTOR	=	C JOHN'S RISK PER 100,000
1. Arteriosclerotic heart disease	723		2.3		1,663
2. Motor vehicle accidents	290		4.5		1,305
3. Suicide	250		1.0		250
4. Cirrhosis	200		2.0		400
5. Homicide	148		1.0		148
6. Lung cancer	141		1.1		155
7. Stroke	106		2.2		233
8. Pneumonia	49		1.0		49
9. Cancer of the large intestine and rectum	44		1.0		44
10. Brain cancer	35		1.0		35
All other causes of death combined	1,214				1,214
				Total	5,496

On the facing page, follow the steps taken by John.

- First, he referred back to the tables on pages 39–52 and learned the number of deaths that can be predicted per 100,000 of his age group in the coming ten years for each of the diseases enumerated. That's column A.
- To fill in column B, his own individual risks, he went back through pages 225 to 259 of this chapter and noted down the risk factors he had calculated for each of the diseases on his list.

YOUR OWN HEALTH PROFILE: Do It Yourself

YOUR SCORE

	A DEATHS PER 100,000	×	B YOUR INDIVIDUAL RISK FACTOR	=	C YOUR RISK PER 100,000
1.					
2.					
3.					
4.					
5.					
6.					
7.					
8.					
9.					
10.					
All other causes of death combined					
				Your Total	

- He got the figures in column C by multiplying the figures in column A by those in column B.
- He added up the numbers of column C, including the number given in his age table for *all other causes of death combined.*

The crucial number is the total at the bottom of column C; take it to the next page with you.

The crucial number computed on page 273 will enable you to discover what your risk age is, as compared with your chronological age. To find your risk age, consult the charts on next four pages.

Here's how: In the "Number of Deaths" column appropriate to you, look first for the number closest to your own total from column C. Then follow across horizontally until you reach the column headed by the last digit of your actual age, and that is your medical risk age.

John finds the number closest to his column C total—5,496—near the top of the chart on page 276 for white males and females. Next he looks at the column headlines, seeking a 7, which is the last digit of his age, 37. When he finds it, he moves his finger down to the right line and discovers that his medical risk age is 42. He's just aged five years.

Thoughtfully, John circles the number. Find and circle your own medical risk age. You might consider using a red pencil if it is five or more years older than your actual age.

HEALTH APPRAISAL AGE TABLES
for white males and females

Find age across from number of deaths closest to patient's total individual risk

Use column headed by figure corresponding to last digit of patient's actual age

WHITE MALE NUMBER OF DEATHS	0 5	1 6	2 7	3 8	4 9	WHITE FEMALE NUMBER OF DEATHS
530	5	6	7	8	9	350
570	6	7	8	9	10	350
630	7	8	9	10	11	350
710	8	9	10	11	12	360
790	9	10	11	12	13	380
880	10	11	12	13	14	410
990	11	12	13	14	15	430
1,110	12	13	14	15	16	460
1,230	13	14	15	16	17	490
1,350	14	15	16	17	18	520
1,440	15	16	17	18	19	550
1,500	16	17	18	19	20	570
1,540	17	18	19	20	21	600
1,560	18	19	20	21	22	620
1,570	19	20	21	22	23	640
1,580	20	21	22	23	24	660
1,590	21	22	23	24	25	690
1,590	22	23	24	25	26	720
1,590	23	24	25	26	27	750
1,600	24	25	26	27	28	790
1,620	25	26	27	28	29	840
1,660	26	27	28	29	30	900
1,730	27	28	29	30	31	970
1,830	28	29	30	31	32	1,040
1,960	29	30	31	32	33	1,130
2,120	30	31	32	33	34	1,220
2,310	31	32	33	34	35	1,330
2,520	32	33	34	35	36	1,460
2,760	33	34	35	36	37	1,600
3,030	34	35	36	37	38	1,760
3,330	35	36	37	38	39	1,930

Find age across from number of deaths closest to patient's total individual risk

Use column headed by figure corresponding to last digit of patient's actual age

WHITE MALE NUMBER OF DEATHS	0 / 5	1 / 6	2 / 7	3 / 8	4 / 9	WHITE FEMALE NUMBER OF DEATHS
3,670	36	37	38	39	40	2,120
4,060	37	38	39	40	41	2,330
4,510	38	39	40	41	42	2,550
5,010	39	40	41	42	43	2,780
5,560	40	41	(42)	43	44	3,020
6,160	41	42	43	44	45	3,280
6,830	42	43	44	45	46	3,560
7,570	43	44	45	46	47	3,870
8,380	44	45	46	47	48	4,220
9,260	45	46	47	48	49	4,600
10,190	46	47	48	49	50	5,000
11,160	47	48	49	50	51	5,420
12,170	48	49	50	51	52	5,860
13,230	49	50	51	52	53	6,330
14,340	50	51	52	53	54	6,850
15,530	51	52	53	54	55	7,440
16,830	52	53	54	55	56	8,110
18,260	53	54	55	56	57	8,870
19,820	54	55	56	57	58	9,730
21,490	55	56	57	58	59	10,680
23,260	56	57	58	59	60	11,720
25,140	57	58	59	60	61	12,860
27,120	58	59	60	61	62	14,100
29,210	59	60	61	62	63	15,450
31,420	60	61	62	63	64	16,930
33,760	61	62	63	64	65	18,560
36,220	62	63	64	65	66	20,360
38,810	63	64	65	66	67	22,340
41,540	64	65	66	67	68	24,520
44,410	65	66	67	68	69	26,920
47,440	66	67	68	69	70	29,560
50,650	67	68	69	70	71	32,470
54,070	68	69	70	71	72	35,690
57,720	69	70	71	72	73	39,250
61,640	70	71	72	73	74	43,200

HEALTH APPRAISAL AGE TABLES
for black males and females

Find age across from number of deaths closest to patient's total individual risk

Use column headed by figure corresponding to last digit of patient's actual age

BLACK MALE NUMBER OF DEATHS	0 5	1 6	2 7	3 8	4 9	BLACK FEMALE NUMBER OF DEATHS
750	5	6	7	8	9	530
810	6	7	8	9	10	540
880	7	8	9	10	11	550
970	8	9	10	11	12	570
1,080	9	10	11	12	13	590
1,210	10	11	12	13	14	630
1,370	11	12	13	14	15	700
1,560	12	13	14	15	16	790
1,760	13	14	15	16	17	890
1,970	14	15	16	17	18	1,000
2,180	15	16	17	18	19	1,110
2,390	16	17	18	19	20	1,240
2,590	17	18	19	20	21	1,370
2,780	18	19	20	21	22	1,510
2,960	19	20	21	22	23	1,660
3,140	20	21	22	23	24	1,810
3,320	21	22	23	24	25	1,970
3,500	22	23	24	25	26	2,140
3,670	23	24	25	26	27	2,320
3,840	24	25	26	27	28	2,520
4,010	25	26	27	28	29	2,720
4,200	26	27	28	29	30	2,930
4,430	27	28	29	30	31	3,150
4,700	28	29	30	31	32	3,390
5,010	29	30	31	32	33	3,650
5,350	30	31	32	33	34	3,920
5,730	31	32	33	34	35	4,210
6,140	32	33	34	35	36	4,530
6,590	33	34	35	36	37	4,880
7,090	34	35	36	37	38	5,260
7,620	35	36	37	38	39	5,670
8,180	36	37	38	39	40	6,100
8,770	37	38	39	40	41	6,540

Find age across from number of deaths closest to patient's total individual risk

Use column headed by figure corresponding to last digit of patient's actual age

BLACK MALE NUMBER OF DEATHS	0 / 5	1 / 6	2 / 7	3 / 8	4 / 9	BLACK FEMALE NUMBER OF DEATHS
9,400	38	39	40	41	42	6,990
10,090	39	40	41	42	43	7,460
10,860	40	41	42	43	44	7,980
11,720	41	42	43	44	45	8,550
12,680	42	43	44	45	46	9,190
13,740	43	44	45	46	47	9,920
14,850	44	45	46	47	48	10,740
15,970	45	46	47	48	49	11,610
17,100	46	47	48	49	50	12,500
18,230	47	48	49	50	51	13,390
19,360	48	49	50	51	52	14,290
20,530	49	50	51	52	53	15,260
21,820	50	51	52	53	54	16,360
23,310	51	52	53	54	55	17,650
25,060	52	53	54	55	56	19,170
27,070	53	54	55	56	57	20,790
29,260	54	55	56	57	58	22,290
31,500	55	56	57	58	59	23,720
33,740	56	57	58	59	60	25,130
35,980	57	58	59	60	61	26,530
38,220	58	59	60	61	62	27,930
40,430	59	60	61	62	63	29,320
42,590	60	61	62	63	64	30,710
44,650	61	62	63	64	65	32,090
46,600	62	63	64	65	66	33,470
48,450	63	64	65	66	67	34,860
50,280	64	65	66	67	68	36,310
52,100	65	66	67	68	69	37,870
53,920	66	67	68	69	70	39,570
55,740	67	68	69	70	71	41,410
57,560	68	69	70	71	72	43,350
59,390	69	70	71	72	73	45,370
61,220	70	71	72	73	74	47,450

Appendix A

WEIGHT TABLES

Desirable weight tables are shown below for adult males and females. The tables assume height and weight taken with shoes and indoor clothing. The first set of tables shows desirable weight ranges for small-frame, medium-frame, and large-frame individuals. The second set of tables shows the percent over or under desirable weight for individuals of medium frame. In using the tables assume that small frame means thin chest, narrow shoulders, and narrow pelvis, and that large frame means thick chest, broad shoulders, and broad pelvis.

DESIRABLE WEIGHTS FOR MEN AND WOMEN AGED 25 AND OVER
(in pounds according to height and frame, in indoor clothing)

MEN

HEIGHT WITH 1-INCH HEELS Feet	Inches	SMALL FRAME	MEDIUM FRAME	LARGE FRAME
5	2	112–120	118–129	126–141
5	3	115–123	121–133	129–144
5	4	118–126	124–136	132–148
5	5	121–129	127–139	135–152
5	6	124–133	130–143	138–156
5	7	128–137	134–147	142–161
5	8	132–141	138–152	147–166
5	9	136–145	142–156	151–170
5	10	140–150	146–160	155–174
5	11	144–154	150–165	159–179
6	0	148–158	154–170	164–184
6	1	152–162	158–175	168–189
6	2	156–167	162–180	173–194
6	3	160–171	167–185	178–199
6	4	164–175	172–190	182–204

APPENDIX A

WOMEN

HEIGHT WITH 2-INCH HEELS		SMALL FRAME	MEDIUM FRAME	LARGE FRAME
Feet	Inches			
4	10	92–98	96–107	104–119
4	11	94–101	98–110	106–122
5	0	96–104	101–113	109–125
5	1	99–107	104–116	112–128
5	2	102–110	107–119	115–131
5	3	105–113	110–122	118–134
5	4	108–116	113–126	121–138
5	5	111–119	116–130	125–142
5	6	114–123	120–135	129–146
5	7	118–127	124–139	133–150
5	8	122–131	128–143	137–154
5	9	126–135	132–147	141–158
5	10	130–140	136–151	145–163
5	11	134–144	140–155	149–168
6	0	138–148	144–159	153–173

Courtesy of Metropolitan Life Insurance Co., New York.

THE LONGEVITY FACTOR

TABLE—PERCENT OVER OR UNDER DESIRABLE WEIGHT FOR MALES

WEIGHT (pounds)	62	63	64	65	66	67	68	69	70	71	72	73	74	75	76
100–104	−17	−20	−22	−23	−25	−27	−30	−32	−33	−35	−37	−39	−40	−42	−44
105–109	−13	−16	−18	−20	−22	−24	−26	−28	−30	−32	−34	−36	−37	−39	−41
110–114	−9	−12	−14	−16	−18	−20	−23	−25	−27	−29	−31	−33	−35	−36	−38
115–119	−5	−8	−10	−12	−14	−17	−19	−21	−24	−26	−28	−30	−32	−34	−35
120–124	0	−4	−6	−8	−11	−13	−16	−18	−20	−23	−25	−27	−29	−31	−33
125–129	3	0	−2	−5	−7	−10	−12	−15	−17	−19	−22	−24	−26	−28	−30
130–134	7	4	0	0	−3	−6	−9	−11	−14	−16	−19	−21	−23	−25	−27
135–139	11	8	5	3	0	−2	−6	−8	−10	−13	−15	−18	−20	−22	−24
140–144	15	12	9	7	4	0	−2	−5	−7	−10	−12	−15	−17	−19	−22
145–149	19	16	13	11	8	5	0	0	−4	−7	−9	−12	−14	−16	−19
150–154	23	20	17	14	11	8	5	2	0	−4	−6	−9	−11	−14	−16
155–159	27	24	21	18	15	12	8	5	3	0	−3	−6	−8	−11	−13
160–164	31	28	25	22	19	15	12	9	6	3	0	−3	−5	−8	−10
165–169	35	31	28	26	22	19	15	12	9	6	3	0	−2	−5	−8
170–174	39	35	32	29	26	22	19	15	12	9	6	3	0	−2	−5
175–179	43	39	36	33	30	26	22	19	16	12	9	6	4	0	−2
180–184	47	43	40	37	33	30	26	22	19	16	12	9	6	3	0
185–189	51	47	44	41	37	33	29	26	22	19	15	12	9	6	3
190–194	55	51	48	44	41	37	32	29	25	22	19	15	12	9	6
195–199	60	55	52	48	44	40	36	32	29	25	22	18	15	12	9
200–204	64	59	55	52	48	44	39	36	32	28	25	21	18	15	12
205–209	68	63	59	56	52	47	43	39	35	31	28	24	21	18	14
210–214	72	67	63	59	55	51	46	42	39	35	31	27	24	20	17
215–219	76	71	67	63	59	54	50	46	42	38	34	30	27	23	20
220–224	80	75	71	67	63	58	53	49	45	41	37	33	30	26	23
225–229	84	79	75	71	66	62	57	52	48	44	40	36	33	29	25
230–234	88	83	78	74	70	65	60	56	52	47	43	39	36	32	28
235–239	92	87	82	78	74	69	63	59	55	50	46	42	39	35	31
240–244	96	91	86	82	77	72	67	62	58	54	49	45	42	37	34
245–249	100	94	90	86	81	76	70	66	61	57	52	48	44	40	36
250–254	……	98	94	89	85	79	74	69	65	60	56	51	47	43	39
255–259	……	100	98	93	88	83	77	72	68	63	59	54	50	46	42
260–264	……	……	100	97	92	86	81	76	71	66	62	57	53	49	45
265–269	……	……	……	100	96	90	84	79	75	70	65	60	56	52	48
270–274	……	……	……	……	99	94	88	83	78	73	68	63	59	55	50
275–279	……	……	……	……	100	97	91	86	81	76	71	66	62	57	53
280–284	……	……	……	……	……	100	94	89	84	79	74	69	65	60	56
285–289	……	……	……	……	……	……	98	93	88	82	77	72	68	63	59
290–294	……	……	……	……	……	……	100	96	91	85	80	75	71	66	61
295–299	……	……	……	……	……	……	……	99	94	89	83	78	74	69	64

HEIGHT (inches)

APPENDIX A

TABLE—PERCENT OVER OR UNDER DESIRABLE WEIGHT FOR FEMALES

WEIGHT (pounds)	58	59	60	61	62	63	64	65	66	67	68	69	70	71	72
80–84	−19	−21	−23	−25	−27	−29	−31	−33	−36	−38	−39	−41	−43	−44	−46
85–89	−14	−16	−19	−21	−23	−25	−27	−29	−32	−34	−36	−38	−39	−41	−43
90–94	−9	−12	−14	−16	−19	−21	−23	−25	−28	−30	−32	−34	−36	−38	−39
95–99	−4	−7	−9	−12	−14	−16	−19	−21	−24	−26	−28	−30	−32	−34	−36
100–104	0	0	−5	−7	−10	−12	−15	−17	−20	−22	−25	−27	−29	−31	−33
105–109	5	3	0	−3	−5	−8	−10	−13	−16	−19	−21	−23	−25	−27	−29
110–114	10	8	5	0	0	−3	−6	−9	−12	−15	−17	−20	−22	−24	−26
115–119	15	12	9	6	4	0	−2	−5	−8	−11	−14	−16	−18	−21	−23
120–124	20	17	14	11	8	5	2	0	−4	−7	−10	−13	−15	−17	−19
125–129	25	22	19	15	12	9	6	3	0	−3	−6	−9	−11	−14	−16
130–134	30	27	23	20	17	14	10	7	4	0	−3	−5	−8	−11	−13
135–139	35	32	28	25	21	18	15	11	7	4	0	−2	−5	−7	−10
140–144	40	37	33	29	26	22	19	15	11	8	5	2	0	−4	−6
145–149	45	41	37	34	30	27	23	20	15	12	8	5	2	0	−3
150–154	50	46	42	38	35	31	27	24	19	16	12	9	6	3	0
155–159	55	51	47	43	39	35	31	28	23	19	16	13	9	6	4
160–164	60	56	51	47	43	40	36	32	27	23	20	16	13	10	7
165–169	65	61	56	52	48	44	40	36	31	27	23	20	16	13	10
170–174	69	65	61	56	52	48	44	40	35	31	27	23	20	17	14
175–179	74	70	65	61	57	53	48	44	39	35	31	27	23	20	17
180–184	79	75	70	65	61	57	52	48	43	38	34	30	27	23	20
185–189	84	80	75	70	65	61	56	52	47	42	38	34	30	27	23
190–194	89	85	79	75	70	66	61	56	51	46	42	38	34	30	27
195–199	94	89	84	79	74	70	65	60	55	50	45	41	37	34	30
200–204	100	94	89	84	79	74	69	64	58	54	49	45	41	37	33
205–209		100	93	88	83	78	73	68	62	57	53	48	44	40	37
210–214			98	93	88	83	77	72	66	61	56	52	48	44	40
215–219			100	97	92	87	82	76	70	65	60	56	51	47	43
220–224				100	96	91	86	80	74	69	64	59	55	51	47
225–229					100	96	90	85	78	73	68	63	58	54	50
230–234						100	94	89	82	76	71	66	62	57	53
235–239							98	93	86	80	75	70	65	61	56
240–244							100	97	90	84	79	73	69	64	60
245–249								100	94	88	82	77	72	67	63

Note: Blanks signify more than 100% overweight.

Source: Based on desirable weights (in ordinary clothing) for men and women of medium frame, at ages 25 and over, according to height (with shoes). Derived from tables in: New weight standards for men and women. Statistical Bulletin, Metropolitan Life Insurance Company 40: p. 3. November–December 1959, which were derived primarily from data of the Build and Blood Pressure Study, 1959, Society of Actuaries.

Appendix B

Here is the complete health profile of Susan Johnson, exactly as it came off the computer of Interhealth of San Diego, to be sent to her:

APPENDIX B

```
JOHNSON, SUSAN          HEALTH RISK PROFILE                         120578
STAYWELL PROGRAM                         DATE  12-05-78  ID  000716327 F
-------------------------------------------------------------------------
CURR B.P.  120/070  PREV B.P. NOT GIVEN CURR CHOL. 203 MG %  PREV CHOL. NOT GIVEN
           HT. 64 IN. WT. 160 LBS. CURR TRIG. 234 MG %  PREV TRIG. NOT GIVEN
-------------------------------------------------------------------------
AVERAGE TEN YEAR RISK OF DEATH PER 100,000       2,892 YOUR PRESENT AGE        40
YOUR CURRENT TEN YEAR RISK OF DEATH PER 100,000  4,393 YOUR CURRENT RISK AGE   46
YOUR ACHIEVABLE TEN YEAR RISK OF DEATH PER 100,000 2,533 YOUR ACHIEVABLE AGE   39
-------------------------------------------------------------------------
AN AVG. WOMAN YOUR AGE HAS  2,852 CHANCES OF DYING PER 100,000 IN THE NEXT 10 YRS.
            YOUR RISKS ARE   54% GREATER THAN THE AVERAGE.
            YOU COULD REDUCE YOUR RISKS BY   42 %.
-------------------------------------------------------------------------
       FACTORS THAT MAY OFFER THE          COMBINED ACHIEVABLE BENEFIT
       GREATEST REDUCTION IN RISK          WITH CHANGE OF THESE FACTORS
           NOT DRINKING................................... 3.0 YRS
           NOT SMOKING.................................... 1.9 YRS
           EXERCISE PROGRAM...............................  .4 YRS
           WEIGHT REDUCTION...............................  .3 YRS
           OTHER.......................................... 1.4 YRS
           TOTAL REDUCTION IN RISK........................ 7.0 YRS
-------------------------------------------------------------------------
           YOUR RISKS IN DESCENDING IMPORTANCE. #1 IS HIGHEST.
   A RISK FACTOR OF 1.0 IS AVERAGE. A RISK FACTOR LESS THAN 1.0 CARRIES LESS THAN
   AVERAGE RISK. A RISK FACTOR ABOVE 1.0 CARRIES GREATER THAN AVERAGE RISK.
-------------------------------------------------------------------------
# 1 ARTERIOSCLEROTIC HEART DISEASE     (HEART ATTACK)
   AVERAGE RISK              308 **********
   YOUR CURRENT RISK         795 **************************          ( 2.6 X AVG)
   YOUR ACHIEVABLE RISK      160 *****                                (  .5 X AVG)

CONTRIBUTING FACTORS   RISK FACTOR   RISK REDUCING FACTORS        RISK FACTOR
B.P. (CURR) ---120/070     .4                                          .4
CHOL (CURR) ---203MG%      .7        CHOLESTEROL 180 OR LESS           .6
DIABETES-NO               1.0                                         1.0
EXERCISE-SEDENTARY        1.4        SUPERVISED EXERCISE              1.0
FH ASHD  ONE PARENT       1.2                                         1.2
SMOKER--2 PACKS/DAY       2.1        NOT SMOKING                       .9
WEIGHT=160 LBS.           1.3        WEIGHT=119 LBS. OR LESS          1.0
NO HX. OF ABNORMAL ECG    1.0                                         1.0
TRIG.---(CUR)---234MG%    1.3        TRIGLYCERIDES < 151 MG%          1.1
EXCESSIVE STRESS MAY INCREASE RISK. EXACT RISK FACTOR NOT YET AVAILABLE.
-------------------------------------------------------------------------
# 2 BREAST CANCER
   AVERAGE RISK              342 **********
   YOUR CURRENT RISK         581 ******************                  ( 1.7 X AVG)
   YOUR ACHIEVABLE RISK      342 **********                          (  AVERAGE )

CONTRIBUTING FACTORS    RISK FACTOR   RISK REDUCING FACTORS       RISK FACTOR
CURRENT FACTOR              1.7       ACHIEVABLE FACTOR               1.0
FAMILY HISTORY=YES
MONTHLY SELF-EXAM=NO                  MONTHLY SELF-EXAM
YEARLY MD EXAM=YES
YEARLY MAMMOGRAPHY=NO                 YEARLY MAMMOGRAPHY
-------------------------------------------------------------------------

           PREPARED BY INTERHEALTH INC. • 2970 5TH AVE., SAN DIEGO, CALIF.
```

THE LONGEVITY FACTOR

```
JOHNSON, SUSAN          HEALTH RISK PROFILE                    (CONTINUED) 120578
STAYWELL PROGRAM                       DATE   12-05-78  ID  000716327 F
---------------------------------------------------------------------------------
# 3 MOTOR VEHICLE ACCIDENTS
  AVERAGE RISK                 93 **********
  YOUR CURRENT RISK           456 *****************************>4.0 ( 4.9 X AVG)
  YOUR ACHIEVABLE RISK         37 ****                              (  .4 X AVG)

  CONTRIBUTING FACTORS   RISK FACTOR    RISK REDUCING FACTORS    RISK FACTOR
  ALCOHOL=25-40 DRINKS/WK   5.0         NONE BEFORE DRIVING          .5
  MILEAGE= 12000            1.0                                     1.0
  SEAT BELTS= 25-74% USE     .9         REGULAR USE OF BELTS         .8
  RX USER=MAY BE FACTOR                 RX=NOT BEFORE DRIVING
---------------------------------------------------------------------------------
# 4 LUNG CANCER
  AVERAGE RISK                149 **********
  YOUR CURRENT RISK           447 *******************************  ( 3.0 X AVG)
  YOUR ACHIEVABLE RISK        358 ************************         ( 2.4 X AVG)

  CONTRIBUTING FACTORS   RISK FACTOR    RISK REDUCING FACTORS    RISK FACTOR
  SMOKER==2 PACKS/DAY       3.0         NOT SMOKING                 2.4
                                        REMAIN STOPPED  6 YEARS      .6
---------------------------------------------------------------------------------
# 5 CIRRHOSIS OF LIVER
  AVERAGE RISK                170 **********
  YOUR CURRENT RISK           425 ****************************     ( 2.5 X AVG)
  YOUR ACHIEVABLE RISK         34 **                                (  .2 X AVG)

  CONTRIBUTING FACTORS   RISK FACTOR    RISK REDUCING FACTORS    RISK FACTOR
  ALCOHOL=25-40 DRINKS/WK   2.5         NOT DRINKING                 .2
  LIVER FUNCTION            1.0                                     1.0
---------------------------------------------------------------------------------
# 6 SUICIDE
  AVERAGE RISK                143 **********
  YOUR CURRENT RISK           143 **********                         ( AVERAGE )
  YOUR ACHIEVABLE RISK        143 **********                         ( AVERAGE )

  CONTRIBUTING FACTORS   RISK FACTOR    RISK REDUCING FACTORS    RISK FACTOR
  NO DEPRESSION             1.0                                     1.0
  FH SUICIDE=NO             1.0                                     1.0
  ALCOHOL=25-40 DRINKS/WK   1.0                                     1.0
---------------------------------------------------------------------------------
# 7 STROKE
  AVERAGE RISK                174 **********
  YOUR CURRENT RISK           136 ********                          (  .8 X AVG)
  YOUR ACHIEVABLE RISK         49 ***                               (  .3 X AVG)

  CONTRIBUTING FACTORS   RISK FACTOR    RISK REDUCING FACTORS    RISK FACTOR
  B.P. (CURR) ==120/070      .4                                      .4
  CHOL (CURR)=== 203MG%      .7                                      .7
  DIABETES=NO               1.0                                     1.0
  SMOKER==2 PACKS/DAY       1.5         NOT SMOKING                 1.0
  NO HX. OF ABNORMAL ECG    1.0                                     1.0
---------------------------------------------------------------------------------

         PREPARED BY INTERHEALTH INC.  •  2970 5TH AVE., SAN DIEGO, CALIF.
```

APPENDIX B

```
JOHNSON, SUSAN          HEALTH RISK PROFILE              (CONTINUED) 120578
STAYWELL PROGRAM                        DATE    12-05-78  ID  000716327 F
------------------------------------------------------------------------
# 8 CANCER OF OVARIES           NO FACTORS FOR THIS CAUSE OF DEATH
    AVERAGE RISK            101 **********
    YOUR CURRENT RISK       101 **********                    ( AVERAGE )
    YOUR ACHIEVABLE RISK    101 **********                    ( AVERAGE )
------------------------------------------------------------------------
# 9 CANCER OF INTESTINES AND RECTUM
    AVERAGE RISK             87 **********
    YOUR CURRENT RISK        87 **********                    ( AVERAGE )
    YOUR ACHIEVABLE RISK     87 **********                    ( AVERAGE )

CONTRIBUTING FACTORS   RISK FACTOR    RISK REDUCING FACTORS   RISK FACTOR
INTESTINAL POLYP-NO        1.0                                    1.0
RECTAL BLEEDING-NO         1.0                                    1.0
ULC. COLITIS- NO           1.0                                    1.0
------------------------------------------------------------------------
#10 CANCER OF CERVIX
    AVERAGE RISK             70 **********
    YOUR CURRENT RISK         7 *                             ( .1 X AVG)
    YOUR ACHIEVABLE RISK      7 *                             ( .1 X AVG)

CONTRIBUTING FACTORS   RISK FACTOR    RISK REDUCING FACTORS   RISK FACTOR
ECONOMIC STATUS-MEDIUM     1.0                                    1.0
INTERCOURSE HX.            1.0                                    1.0
PAP 3 NEG IN 5 YEARS        .1           ANNUAL IN FUTURE          .1
------------------------------------------------------------------------
OTHER: ALL OTHER CAUSES OF DEATH (APPROX 1000) WHOSE TOTAL RISK IS  1,215
------------------------------------------------------------------------
    THIS APPRAISAL IS BASED ON POSSIBLE 10 YEAR RISK USING DATA BELIEVED TO BE VALID.
PRE-EXISTING DISEASE MAY TOTALLY INVALIDATE THE RESULT. THE RISK REDUCING MEASURES
HOWEVER ARE ONLY GUIDELINES FOR THE INDIVIDUAL AND SHOULD BE UNDERTAKEN ONLY WITH
THE SUPERVISION OF A PHYSICIAN. THE 1974 GELLER TABLES ARE UTILIZED IN
THE COMPUTATIONS. RISK FACTORS ARE CONSTANTLY APPRAISED AND UPDATED AS DATA WARRANTS
```

PREPARED BY INTERHEALTH INC. • 2970 5TH AVE., SAN DIEGO, CALIF.

Index

Abortions, death rate from complications of, by age and race, 40–43
Accidents
 death rate from, by age, sex, and race, 39–52
 See also specific types of accidents
Addresses of centers using health profiling, 201–2
Age
 death rates among men and women, by race and, 39–52
 health appraisal tables by sex, race, and, 275–78
Age expectancy, 16
Aircraft accidents
 death rate from, by age, sex, and race, 42–44
 in Garro case, 176
Alcohol consumption, 35
 and auto accidents, 36
 in Blake case, 80–82
 and cancer, 35
 cross-addiction to drugs and alcohol, 141
 in Eastman case, 169
 in Garro case, 175, 176
 in Howell case, 96, 98, 100
 in Johnson case, 18, 23, 287, 288
 in Mooney case, 144–46
 questionnaire on, 198
 in your own profile, 210–11, 236–38, 240–42, 244–45, 254–255
 See also Cirrhosis of the liver
Alcoholics Anonymous, 62–63, 134–38, 140–41, 189
Alcoholism
 cases illustrating alchoholism, 55–66, 128–43
 cases illustrating alcoholism, health profiles of, 66–71, 144–147
 death rate from, by age, sex, and race, 43–47
Aleukemia in Mooney case, 146
Aluminum Company of America (ALCOA), 218–19
American Heart Association, 151, 154
Andrew, Fred W., 219, 220
Anemias
 death rate from, by age, sex, and race, 39
 sickle cell, 206
Arrests, *see* Violence
Arterial diseases
 in Eastman case, 169
 in Howell case, 99
 in your own profile, 267–68

INDEX

Arteriosclerotic heart disease
  in Blake case, 82
  death rate from, by age, sex, and race, 42–52
  in Eastman case, 167
  in Garro case, 177
  in Hanson case, 67
  in Howell case, 96–97
  in Johnson case, 21–22, 287
  in your own profile, 226–35, 272–73
Asbestos, respiratory diseases and, 37
Asthma, smoking and, 37
Attitudes
  and changing habits, 186–87
  health and, 159–66
Arizona, University of, 28–29
Automobile accidents, *see* Motor vehicle accidents

Backsliding in old habits, 191–93
Bacterial pneumonia, *see* Pneumonia
Benson, Herbert, M.D., 185
Birth control pills
  in Blake case, 83
  in your own profile, 215
Bladder cancer, death rate from, by age, sex, and race, 52
Blake, Laura (case history), 72–79, 189
  health profile of, 79–84
Blood pressure
  in Blake case, 82
  cardiovascular disease and, 34
  in Eastman case, 167–70
  in Garro case, 174, 177, 178
  habit change and, 31
  in Hanson case, 67, 69

  in Howell case, 96–99
  in Johnson case, 21, 287
  in Kodaly case, 157
  in Meeker case, 111–13
  in Mooney case, 146
  in your own profile, 206, 216, 230–35, 250–52, 264–65, 267–269
Blue Cross, 29
Brain cancer
  death rate from, by age, sex, and race, 39–41
  in Garro case, 177
  in Mooney case, 147
  in your own profile, 258–59, 272–73
Breast cancer
  in Blake case, 80
  death rate from, by age, sex, and race, 42–52
  in Eastman case, 168–69
  in Johnson case, 22
  in Meeker case, 112
  in your own profile, 214, 260
Brethauer, Edgar, Jr., M.D., 218–219
Bronchitis
  death rate from, by age, sex, and race, 48–52
  in Eastman case, 170
  in Howell case, 98
  smoking and chronic, 37

Cancer
  attitude and, 160–61, 164–65
  risk of, 34–35
  smoking and, 34–35
  and your own profile, 213
  See also specific types of cancer

INDEX

Carcinogens, 35n
Cardiovascular disease
  risk of, 34
  See also Arterial diseases;
    Arteriosclerotic heart
    disease; Heart disease;
    Hypertensive heart disease
Center for Disease Control
  (HEW), 218
Central nervous system, cancer of
  in Garro case, 177
  in Mooney case, 147
Cervical cancer
  in Blake case, 83-84
  death rate from, by age and
    race, 44-50
  in Meeker case, 115
  in your own profile, 214-15,
    261-62
Checkups, periodic, habit change
    and, 30, 31
Chemicals, carcinogenic, 35
Cholesterol levels
  in Blake case, 82
  cardiovascular disease and high
    serum, 34
  in Eastman case, 167-69
  in Garro case, 177-78
  in Hanson case, 67, 69
  in Howell case, 97-99
  in Johnson case, 21, 287, 288
  in Kodaly case, 157
  in Meeker case, 111, 112
  in Mooney case, 146
  reducing intake of cholesterol,
    30
  in Solomon case, 122-23, 126
  in your own profile, 216, 228-
    229, 232-36, 248-49, 253,
    267, 268
Cigarette smoking, *see* Smoking

Cirrhosis of the liver, 34, 35-36
  in Blake case, 80
  death rate from, by age, sex,
    and race, 42-51
  in Hanson case, 70
  in Howell case, 98
  incidence of, 35-36
  in Johnson case, 23, 288
  in Meeker case, 114
  in your own profile, 210-11,
    242-43, 272-73
Computers, 17
  in health profiling, 201-2, 218
  and questionnaire on health,
    203-17
Congenital circulatory defects,
  death rate from, by age, sex,
    and race, 39-41
  in Mooney case, 147
Congenital heart defects
  death rate from, by age, sex,
    and race, 39
Cost of medical care, 26
Cystic fibrosis, death rate
  from, by age, sex, and race, 39

Daedalus (magazine), 26
Death
  causes of, 38
  Geller-Steele tables on causes
    of, 39-52
Death rate
  from cirrhosis of the liver in the
    United Kingdom, 36
  from diabetes, 37
  in health appraisal age tables,
    275-78
Death risk
  in Blake case, 79, 84
  in Eastman case, 167, 171
  in Garro case, 174, 178

INDEX

Death risk (*cont.*)
  in Hanson case, 66, 71
  in Howell case, 96, 100
  in Johnson case, 18–19, 21, 287, 289
  in Meeker case, 110, 115
  in Mooney case, 143, 144, 147
  in your own profile, 225, 272–74
Degenerative diseases
  natural history of, 31–32
  preventing, 16
  See also specific degenerative diseases
Depression
  in Blake case, 81
  in Garro case, 175
  in Hanson case, 68
  in Howell case, 100
  in Johnson case, 288
  in Mooney case, 145
  suicide and, 36; *see also* Suicide
  in your own profile, 240–41
Diabetes, 37
  in Blake case, 82, 83
  and cardiovascular disease, 34
  death rate from, by age, sex, and race, 42, 43
  in Eastman case, 167–69
  in Garro case, 177, 178
  in Hanson case, 67, 69
  in Howell case, 97–99
  in Johnson case, 21, 288
  in Meeker case, 111, 112
  in Mooney case, 147
  in your own profile, 205, 217, 228–29, 248–49, 266
"Doing Better and Feeling Worse: Health in the United States" (Knowles), 26
Dreaming, alcoholism and cessation of, 63

Drinking, *see* Alcohol consumption
Driving, *see* Mileage
Drownings
  death rate from, by age, sex, and race, 39–44
  in Mooney case, 147
Drugs
  and auto accidents, 36
  cross-addiction to alcohol and, 141
  questionnaire on, 198
  in your own profile, 210
Dunton, Sabina, 29

Eastman, Emily (case history), 159–66
  health profile of, 166–71
Eating
  case illustrating overeating, 101–10
  case illustrating overeating, health profile of, 110–15
  disease and habits in, 38
  questionnaire on nutrition, 198
  See also Weight
Economic status
  in Blake case, 72
  in Johnson case, 289
  in Meeker case, 102
  in your own profile, 204
Electrocardiograms
  in Blake case, 83
  in Eastman case, 167, 168
  in Garro case, 177, 178
  in Hanson case, 67, 69
  in Howell case, 97, 98
  in Johnson case, 287
  in Meeker case, 111, 112
  in Solomon case, 118
  in your own profile, 206, 217

Emphysema
  death rate from, by age, sex, and race, 47–52
  in Eastman case, 169, 170
  in Garro case, 176
  in Hanson case, 70
  in Howell case, 98, 100
  in Meeker case, 113
  in Mooney case, 146
  smoking and, 37
  in your own profile, 208, 254–255, 269
Environmental exposure, 38
Esophagus, cancer of, death rate from, by age, sex, and race, 47–49
Examination (self-examination; physicians' examination)
  in Blake case, 80
  in Johnson case, 22, 287
  in Meeker case, 112
  in your own profile, 214, 260
Exercise
  in Blake case, 82
  cardiovascular disease and, 34
  disease and, 38
  in Eastman case, 167
  in Garro case, 177
  habit change and, 30, 31
  in Hanson case, 67
  in Howell case, 97
  in Johnson case, 21, 287
  in Kodaly case, 154
  in Meeker case, 111
  questionnaire on, 198
  in Solomon case, 121, 123, 124
  in your own profile, 205, 226–227, 232
Exploration, as stage in process of changing habits, 182–88

Fallat, Robert J., M.D., 157–58
Falls
  death rate from, by age, sex, and race, 40–42, 46
  in Garro case, 177
Family history
  of alcoholism in Hanson case, 55
  of angina in Solomon case, 116
  of arteriosclerotic heart disease in your own profile, 226–27, 232, 234
  of breast cancer in Blake case, 80
  of breast cancer in Johnson case, 22
  of breast cancer in Meeker case, 112
  of breast cancer in your own profile, 260
  cardiovascular disease and, 34
  of diabetes in your own profile, 205, 266
  health and, 172–74
  of heart disease in Blake case, 82
  of heart disease in Eastman case, 167
  of heart disease in Howell case, 97
  of heart disease in Johnson case, 22, 287
  of heart disease in Kodaly case, 149
  of heart disease in Meeker case, 111
  of heart disease in your own profile, 205
  of suicide in Blake case, 81
  of suicide in Garro case, 175
  of suicide in Hanson case, 68

INDEX

Family history (*cont.*)
  of suicide in Howell case, 100
  of suicide in Johnson case, 288
  of suicide in Mooney case, 145
  of suicide in your own profile, 240–41
Females, *see* Women
Fire, death rate from, by age, sex, and race, 39–42
Firearm accidents
  death rate from, by age, sex, and race, 39–42
  See also Violence
Ford Motor Company, 219
Framingham study, 28

Garro, Claudia (wife), 172–73
Garro, James F. (case history), 172–74
  profile of, 174–78
Geller, Harvey, 33
Geller-Steele tables (Geller tables), 33, 38–52
General Health, 201
Groups, joining, 189–90

Habits, changing of, 30–31, 181–193
Hall, Jack H., M.D., 28
Hanson, Donald (case history), 55–66, 189
  profile of, 66–71
Health appraisal age tables, 275–278
Health profiling (Health Hazard Appraisal; Health Risk Analysis; Health Risk Profile), 16–17
  addresses of centers using, 201–202
  computer-assisted, 201–2, 218
  computer-assisted, questionnaire, 203–17
  development of, 28–32
  Institute of Health Research and, 156
  short form, of, 198–200
  tables basic to, 33, 38–52, 275–278; *see also* Weight tables
  your own form for, 223–25, 226–74
Heart disease
  costs of, 26
  death rate from, of U.S. males, 34
  diabetes and, 37
  Framingham study on, 28
  and overeating, case illustrating, 116–27
  See also Arteriosclerotic heart disease; Hypertensive heart disease; Rheumatic heart disease
Heart murmur in your own profile, 270
Hodgkin's disease, death rate from, by age, sex, and race, 42
Homicide, 34, 36
  death rate from, by age, sex, and race, 39–50
  in Garro case, 175
  in Hanson case, 68–69
  in Meeker case, 113
  in Mooney case, 145
  in your own profile, 244–45, 272–73
How to Practice Prospective Medicine (Robbins and Hall), 28

INDEX

Howell, Eugene (case history), 85–95, 193
  profile of, 96–100
Howell, Suzanne (wife), 86–94
Hughes, Lewis, 29
Hydrocephalus, death rate from, by age, sex, and race, 39
Hylinski, Ralph, M.D., 186
Hypertensive heart disease
  death rate from, by age, sex, and race, 44–52
  in Eastman case, 170
  in Meeker case, 113
  in your own profile, 264–65
Hypnosis, 186–87

Institute of Health Research (University of California), 148–49, 153, 156, 157
Institute for Life Style Improvement, 201
Interhealth, 201, 202, 220
Intestinal cancer
  in Blake case, 81–82
  death rate from, by age, sex, and race, 45–52
  in Eastman case, 168
  in Hanson case, 69
  in Howell case, 99
  in Johnson case, 289
  in your own profile, 256–57, 272–73
Intestinal polyps
  in Blake case, 81
  in Eastman case, 168
  in Hanson case, 69
  in Howell case, 99
  in Johnson case, 289
  in your own profile, 208, 256–57

Johnson, Samuel, 92
Johnson, Susan (case history), 18–20
  profile of, 21–24, 286–89

Kellogg Foundation, W. K., 29
Kimberly Clark (paper company), 219
Knowles, John, M.D., 26–27
Kodaly, Jack (case history), 148–158, 184

LaDou, Joseph, M.D., 29
Leukemia
  death rate from, by age, sex, and race, 39–43
  in Mooney case, 146
Lung cancer
  in Blake case, 81
  death rate from, by age, sex, and race, 44–52
  in Eastman case, 169–70
  in Hanson case, 67–68
  in Howell case, 97
  in Johnson case, 23, 288
  in Meeker case, 114
  natural history of, 31–32
  ten-year risk of death from, table, 95
  treatment of, 89–92
  among women, 79
  in your own profile, 246–47, 272–73

Machine-related accidents (excluding cars),
  death rate from, by age, sex, and race, 39–46
  in Garro case, 176
  in Hanson case, 70
Males, *see* Men

INDEX

Mammography in Johnson case, 22, 287
Marijuana, and auto accidents, 36
Medical Datamation, 201
Meditation, 174, 185
Meeker, Lucille (case history), 101–10, 189*n*, 191
    profile of, 110–15
Meeker, Wayne (husband), 102, 107–8
Men
    death rate among, by race and age, 39–52
    health appraisal age tables, by race, 275–88
    percent over or under desirable weight, table, 282
    weight table for, 280
Methodist Hospital of Indiana, 202
Mileage
    in Blake case, 82
    in Garro case, 175
    in Hanson case, 68
    in Johnson case, 18, 23, 287, 288
    in Mooney case, 144
    questionnaire on, 199
    in your own profile, 209, 236–39
Mooney, Kathleen (case history), 128–43, 189, 193
    profile of, 144–47
Mooney, Paul (husband), 132–34
Motor vehicle accidents, 34, 36
    in Blake case, 82
    death rate from, by age, sex, and race, 39–49
    in Garro case, 174–75
    in Hanson case, 68
    in Johnson case, 22–23, 288
    in Mooney case, 144
    in your own profile, 209, 236–239, 272–73

National Aeronautics and Space Administration (NASA), health profiling at, 29
National Cancer Institute, 35
Nephritis and nephrosis
    death rate from, by age, sex, and race, 46, 48–50, 52
    in Meeker case, 114
"Normal" health, changing habits and, 148–58
Nutrition, questionnaire on, 198

Ovarian cancer
    in Blake case, 81
    death rate from, by age and race, 45–52
    in Eastman case, 170
    in Johnson case, 289

Palomar College, 29
Pap smear test
    in Blake case, 84
    in Johnson case, 289
    in Meeker case, 115
    in your own profile, 215, 262
Personal health, questionnaire on, 199
Physicians, examination by, *see* Examination
Pledging of changes in habits, 30–31
Pneumonia
    death rate from, by age, sex, and race, 39–52
    in Eastman case, 169
    in Garro case, 176
    in Hanson case, 70
    in Howell case, 99–100

INDEX

in Meeker case, 113
in Mooney case, 145-46
smoking and, 37
in your own profile, 208, 254-255, 272-73
Poisonings
　death rate from, by age, sex, and race, 40-44
　in Mooney case, 146
Pregnancy, death rate from complications in, by age and race, 40-43
Preventive medicine, as approach to medicine, 25-28
Pritikin, Nathan, 120-24
Pritikin Clinic, 120-22, 189
Prostate cancer
　death rate from, by age and race, 49-52
　in Howell case, 100
Public Health Service, 27, 28

Race
　death rate by age, sex, and, 39-52
　health appraisal age tables by age, sex, and, 275-78
Rectal bleeding
　in Blake case, 82
　in Eastman case, 168
　in Hanson case, 69
　in Howell case, 99
　in Johnson case, 289
　in your own profile, 208, 256-57
Rectal cancer
　in Blake case, 81-82
　death rate from, by age, sex, and race, 45-52
　in Eastman case, 168
　in Hanson case, 69
　in Howell case, 99

in Johnson case, 289
in your own profile, 208-09, 256-57, 272-73
Relaxation Response, The (Benson), 185
Respiratory diseases, 34, 36-37
　See also specific respiratory diseases
Rheumatic heart disease
　death rate from, by age, sex, and race, 41, 42, 48-51
　in your own profile, 206, 270
Road and water safety, questionnaire on, 199
Robbins, Lewis C., M.D., 27-28, 31-33
Ross, Charles M., M.D., 166, 220-22

Sears, Roebuck & Company, 219
Seat belt use
　and auto accidents, 36
　in Blake case, 82
　in Garro case, 175
　and habit change, 30, 31
　in Hanson case, 68
　in Johnson case, 23, 288
　in Mooney case, 144
　in your own profile, 209, 236-39
Self-examination, *see* Examination
Sentry Insurance, 219
Seventh-Day Adventists clinics, 191
Sex
　death rate by age, race, and, 39-52
　health appraisal age tables, by race and, 275-78
　See also Men; Women

INDEX

Sexual intercourse
   in Blake case, 84
   in Johnson case, 289
   in Meeker case, 115
   in your own profile, 215, 261
Sherwood, John N., M.D., 29
Sickle cell anemia, 206
Sigmoidoscopy
   in Eastman case, 168
   in Howell case, 99
   in your own profile, 208, 256-57
Smokenders, 75-77, 189
Smoking (tobacco)
   in Blake case, 81, 82
   cancer and, 34-35
   as carcinogenic, 35
   cardiovascular disease and, 34-35
   cases illustrating, health profiles, 79-84, 96-100
   changing habit of, 30, 31, 183, 184, 186, 191, 192
   degenerative diseases and, 31, 32
   disease and, 38
   in Eastman case, 169, 170
   in Garro case, 177, 178
   in Hanson case, 67, 68
   in Howell case, 96-100
   in Johnson case, 18, 21-23, 287, 288
   in Mooney case, 144, 146, 147
   "normal" health and, 151-55
   and other contaminants, 37
   questionnaire on, 198-99
   respiratory diseases and, 37
   risk of death from lung cancer and, table, 95
   in your own profile, 207, 226-227, 232, 234-35, 246-49, 252-55, 267-69

Society of Prospective Medicine, 28, 201
Solomon, Ed (case history), 116-127, 189
Spiegel, David, M.D., 188*n*
Spiegel, Herbert, M.D., 186-88
Stomach cancer, death rate from, by age, sex, and race, 48-52
Stress
   in Blake case, 83
   controlling, 30
   in Hanson case, 67
   in Howell case, 97
   in Meeker case, 111
Stroke
   in Blake case, 83
   death rate from, by age, sex, and race, 39-52
   diabetes and, 37
   in Eastman case, 168
   in Garro case, 178
   in Hanson case, 69
   in Howell case, 97-98
   in Johnson case, 288
   in Meeker case, 112
   in Mooney case, 146-47
   in your own profile, 217, 248-253, 272-73
Sugar, per capita consumption of refined, 37
Suicide, 34, 36
   in Blake case, 80-81
   death rate from, by age, sex, and race, 40-50
   in Garro case, 175
   in Hanson case, 68
   in Howell case, 100
   in Johnson case, 288
   in Mooney case, 145
   in your own profile, 211-13, 240-41, 272-73

INDEX

Superior Farms (subsidiary of Superior Oil Company), 219

Trance and Treatment—Clinical Uses of Hypnosis (Spiegel and Spiegel), 188*n*
Transcendental Meditation, 174
Triglyceride levels
  in Blake case, 83
  in Eastman case, 167
  in Garro case, 177
  in Hanson case, 67
  in Howell case, 97
  in Johnson case, 22, 287
  in Kodaly case, 157
  in Meeker case, 111
  in your own profile, 216
Tuberculosis in your own profile, 208

Ulcerative colitis
  in Blake case, 82
  in Eastman case, 168
  in Hanson case, 69
  in Howell case, 99
  in your own profile, 209, 256–57
United Kingdom, cirrhosis of the liver in, incidence, 36
Uterine cancer
  death rate from, by age and race, 51
  in your own profile, 214, 263

Violence
  in Garro case, 175
  in Hanson case, 69
  homicide and, 36; *see also* Homicide
  in Meeker case, 113
  in Mooney case, 145
  in your own profile, 244–45
  See also Suicide; Weapons, carrying of

Warner, H. Lynn, 29–31
Water safety, questionnaire on, 199
Water transportation accidents, death rate from, by age, sex, and race, 41
Weapon, carrying of
  in Garro case, 175
  in Hanson case, 69
  in Meeker case, 113
  in Mooney case, 145
  in your own profile, 213, 244–45
Weight
  in Blake case, 83
  cardiovascular disease and, 34
  diabetes and, 37
  in Eastman case, 167, 170
  in Garro case, 177
  habit change and loss of, 30
  in Hanson case, 67
  in Howell case, 96, 97
  in Johnson case, 21, 22, 287
  in Kodaly case, 157
  in Meeker case, 110, 111, 113
  in your own profile, 203, 228–229, 264–66
Weight tables, 280–81
  determining percent over or under desirable weight, 282–283
Weight Watchers, 103, 190
Wellness Resources Center, 202
Williams, George, M.D., 149, 151, 157
Women
  death rate among, by race and age, 39–52

INDEX

Women (*cont.*)
  health appraisal age tables, by race, 275–78
  lung cancer among, 79
  percent over or under desirable weight, table, 283
  weight table for, 281